BMAT and UKCAT
Uncovered

Dedication

To our parents
for life, love and learning

Acknowledgements

We would like to thank:

Our teachers for inspiring us; Karen Sayal and our students for their valuable feedback; Russ Daff for his illustrations;

Ian Stannard and Paul Maddren at Christs Hospital for support and encouragement; Mary Banks and her team at Wiley-Blackwell.

BMAT and UKCAT Uncovered

A guide to medical school entrance exams

BY

T. O. Osinowo

R. A. Weerakkody

H. W. Woodward

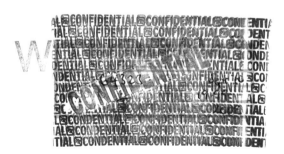

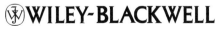

WILEY-BLACKWELL

A John Wiley & Sons, Ltd., Publication

BMJ|Books

This edition first published 2008, © 2008 by T. O. Osinowo, R. A. Weerakkody, H. W. Woodward

BMJ Books is an imprint of BMJ Publishing Group Limited, used under licence by Blackwell Publishing which was acquired by John Wiley & Sons in February 2007. Blackwell's publishing programme has been merged with Wiley's global Scientific, Technical and Medical business to form Wiley-Blackwell.

Registered office: John Wiley & Sons Ltd, The Atrium, Southern Gate, Chichester, West Sussex, PO19 8SQ, UK

Editorial offices: 9600 Garsington Road, Oxford, OX4 2DQ, UK
The Atrium, Southern Gate, Chichester, West Sussex, PO19 8SQ, UK
111 River Street, Hoboken, NJ 07030-5774, USA

For details of our global editorial offices, for customer services and for information about how to apply for permission to reuse the copyright material in this book please see our website at www.wiley.com/wiley-blackwell

The right of the author to be identified as the author of this work has been asserted in accordance with the Copyright, Designs and Patents Act 1988.

Wiley also publishes its books in a variety of electronic formats. Some content that appears in print may not be available in electronic books.

Designations used by companies to distinguish their products are often claimed as trademarks. All brand names and product names used in this book are trade names, service marks, trademarks or registered trademarks of their respective owners. The publisher is not associated with any product or vendor mentioned in this book. This publication is designed to provide accurate and authoritative information in regard to the subject matter covered. It is sold on the understanding that the publisher is not engaged in rendering professional services. If professional advice or other expert assistance is required, the services of a competent professional should be sought.

The contents of this work are intended to further general scientific research, understanding, and discussion only and are not intended and should not be relied upon as recommending or promoting a specific method, diagnosis, or treatment by physicians for any particular patient. The publisher and the author make no representations or warranties with respect to the accuracy or completeness of the contents of this work and specifically disclaim all warranties, including without limitation any implied warranties of fitness for a particular purpose. In view of ongoing research, equipment modifications, changes in governmental regulations, and the constant flow of information relating to the use of medicines, equipment, and devices, the reader is urged to review and evaluate the information provided in the package insert or instructions for each medicine, equipment, or device for, among other things, any changes in the instructions or indication of usage and for added warnings and precautions. Readers should consult with a specialist where appropriate. The fact that an organization or Website is referred to in this work as a citation and/or a potential source of further information does not mean that the author or the publisher endorses the information the organization or Website may provide or recommendations it may make. Further, readers should be aware that Internet Websites listed in this work may have changed or disappeared between when this work was written and when it is read. No warranty may be created or extended by any promotional statements for this work. Neither the publisher nor the author shall be liable for any damages arising herefrom.

Library of Congress Cataloging-in-Publication Data

Osinowo, T. O.
 BMAT and UKCAT uncovered : a guide to medical school entrance exams / by T. O. Osinowo, R. A. Weerakkody, H. W. Woodward
   p. ; cm.
 Includes bibliographical references and index.
 ISBN: 978-1-4051-6918-9
 1. UK Clinical Aptitude Test—Study guides. 2. BioMedical Admissions Test—Study guides.
I. Weerakkody, R. A. II. Woodward, H. W. (Harry W.) III. Title.
 [DNLM: 1. Schools, Medical—Great Britain—Examination Questions. 2. Education,
Medical—Great Britain—Examination Questions. 3. School Admission Criteria—Great Britain—
Examination Questions. W 18.2 O82b 2008]
 R838.5.O85 2008
 610.71'141—dc22   2008023444

A catalogue record for this book is available from the British Library.

Set in Meridien 9.5/12 by Charon Tec Ltd., A Macmillan Company.
Printed in Singapore by Markono Print Media Pte Ltd

3   2010

Contents

Foreword

Selecting students for a medical school education is, perhaps understandably, very difficult. Medicine is a multi-faceted challenging activity requiring considerable intellectual and practical competencies as well as interpersonal skills. UK medical schools are conscious of the fact that to cope with the demands of their medical courses and subsequently become effective doctors, prospective students need to be of high intelligence and come equipped with nimble problem-solving minds. There has been a perception amongst those selecting prospective medical students that even the ability to get top grades in A level examinations is not a sufficient discriminator with which to choose students of sufficient intellectual ability to interview (when their interpersonal skills can be judged). Hence the development over the last 10 years of the BMAT and UKCAT exams by medical schools in the United Kingdom and others such as the GAMSAT in Australia.

These exams are designed to test prospective medical students' intellectual ability, quickness of thinking and reasoning ability in a manner that is relevant to their future work as doctors and their ability to cope with a lengthy and often demanding medical course. Proper preparation for these exams is essential, not because an unsuitable candidate can thus pass the test but to ensure that a student who is capable does not fall at this first hurdle because he or she did not know what to expect. This book cannot replace all the hard work at school that is required to get good GCSE grades and A levels but should be invaluable in going the further mile that is required for medical school entry. Who better to guide prospective students in this than the authors of this book, only recently faced with both the tests and the subsequent rigours (and joys) of the medical course in Cambridge?

I can commend this book to all those who are facing medical school entrance exams and need the excellent guidance and thorough preparation which the three authors provide. This should enable a prospective student of sufficient cognitive ability to pass this hurdle and thence pursue what many in it consider the most satisfying career possible, that is the combination of scientific knowledge with practical and interpersonal skills to solve the problems of disease and illness.

Dr Chris Allen MA MD FRCP
Consultant Neurologist & previous Clinical Dean (1996–2003)
University of Cambridge School of Clinical Medicine

Preface

When applying to medical school, we were startled to hear that we had to take a new test which was different to anything we had taken before. This test, a pilot version of the BMAT, was different because the questions tested how you actually thought and applied knowledge rather than the knowledge itself. It was quite unfamiliar, up until then we had been in the habit of having a syllabus and past questions for every exam we sat. Unfortunately, apart from a few sample questions on the official website, there wasn't much we could do to prepare for this new test. Needless to say, we were scared because we felt unprepared for a test in which we wanted to do our best.

Since then, medical school entrance exams like the BMAT and UKCAT have been rolled out to cover most medical schools, some vet schools and some biomedical courses across the country. The same fear of the unknown which we felt so clearly is apparent in students today, because even now it is very difficult to prepare: after diligently scouring the internet students finds themselves at a loss as to what will come up and how to go about answering the questions. However, it is obvious that after initially familiarising themselves with the format of the questions and developing a systematic approach they find they feel more comfortable and do much better.

It is therefore one of the aims of this book to unravel the basics of these exams, and to show you how it is possible to approach them effectively with only basic knowledge.

The other more obvious objective is to prepare you for the exams, not by teaching tricks or gimmicks but by actually attempting to make you a better thinker. As a result although this book is written with the average applicant to the top medical schools in mind, it is suitable for any student of Thinking Skills.

But this book cannot be relied on as the only thing you need to help you with these tests. It is meant to serve as a kick-start or springboard to set you on a journey of exercising your thinking faculties. This has several implications:

1 You should read the whole book cover-to-cover several times over, regardless of which exam you intend to sit. You are advised to do this because many of the more subtle points are easily missed on first approach.
2 Because this book is about Thinking Skills, conventional rote-learning approaches will not work: to get the best, you have to think. It is created to be more of a workbook than a textbook, with questions and sugges-

tions to pique your interest and stimulate thought. Many questions in the book remain unanswered: the reason for this is to stimulate discussion and debate, using the book with your friends and teachers.

3 This also means that you will need and should want to go beyond this book, searching for other resources, and expanding the quality of the practice you acquire. So the earlier you read and digest this book, the better. You may find visiting our website www.cambridgethinking.com helpful.

What is the BMAT?

The BMAT (Biomedical Admissions Test) is a 2-hour exam composed of three sections introduced by several medical schools, including Cambridge, Oxford, Imperial College, University College London and the Royal Veterinary College, which tests:

- Section 1 (60 minutes): Problem solving and data handling, critical thinking and comprehension.
- Section 2 (30 minutes): Scientific knowledge (the core syllabuses of GCSE science and maths) with a focus on its application, rather than factual recall.
- Section 3 (30 minutes): Written communication in response to a stimulus question.

What is the UKCAT?

The UKCAT (United Kingdom Clinical Aptitude Test) is a 2-hour exam introduced by the majority of the other medical schools in the United Kingdom. It is administered in test centres around the country and is computer based. The sections of the UKCAT are:

- Verbal Reasoning (22 minutes): Comprehension and inference.
- Quantitative Reasoning (22 minutes): Calculations and data handling.
- Abstract Reasoning (16 minutes): Spatial problem solving.
- Decision Analysis (30 minutes): Decoding and encoding messages.
- Non-Cognitive Analysis (30 minutes): Psychometric test in a questionnaire style.

These serve as a summary, and you are encouraged to look at the official websites for both these tests for the latest up to date information.

How to use the book

The layout of the book has been chosen to allow ease of use. There are four main sections:

1 The core two chapters cover numeracy and verbal skills required by every candidate.

2 The BMAT-specific chapters cover Sections 2 and 3 of the BMAT.

3 The UKCAT-specific chapters cover Abstract Reasoning and Decision Analysis for the UKCAT.

4 The Question Papers for the BMAT and UKCAT.

Candidates who wish to prepare exclusively for either the BMAT alone or the UKCAT alone need only read the core two chapters plus the sections relevant to their exam, but we believe you will gain even more by reading the whole book irrespective of which exam you are sitting.

Finally, although this book is primarily aimed at prospective medical and veterinary school applicants, the Thinking Skills required for the BMAT and UKCAT are increasingly becoming a requirement in many other tests (e.g. the LNAT for prospective lawyers, the TSA for prospective computer scientists and even tests by graduate recruiters for large corporate employers) as well as life in general. This book may therefore have a wider forum.

Enjoy!

T. O. Osinowo

R. A. Weerakkody

H.W. Woodward

www.cambridgethinking.com

CHAPTER 1

Quantitative analysis for the BMAT and the UKCAT

Part A: First glance

Problem solving is an essential and common skill. In everyday life, it is a process that makes us stop and think because it is a skill that usually involves deriving new knowledge or information from what we already know or have. In the context of the BMAT and UKCAT we are provided with novel problems and scenarios (usually involving quantitative data) where prior knowledge alone is insufficient. It is the analysis required to be able to derive a solution from the quantitative data that this chapter aims to cover.

There are various steps involved in solving problems of this kind. Firstly you must pick out the relevant information from all the information you have been provided, then you must *think* and decide how to go about using this data to achieve the solution; finally you then go ahead and manipulate the data, drawing on basic *understanding* and *experience* of how the world works, leading to your solution.

Data $\longrightarrow$ Extract relevant data $\longrightarrow$ Determine optimum strategy for achieving solution $\longrightarrow$ Manipulate data appropriately (apply basic skills/functions) $\longrightarrow$ Solution.

Different types of problems give emphasis to different parts of this process. Some problems will require you to decide on the most relevant data in a situation and not much else while others will test the whole range of sub-skills.

Part of this process of problem solving is usually done automatically and is arguably best left that way. What you can do to improve speed and accuracy is consider the tools commonly used in solving problems; the kind of information you will be given and the basic skills and functions you have available in order to manipulate the available data. In this vein, this chapter looks at the various functions that underpin problem solving. These functions are the basic abilities everyone is presumed to have in order to be able to solve problems. Some are very basic indeed and are covered very early in formal education but it is exactly this fact – that they are basic – that seems to be the undoing of many candidates. Getting a firm grasp of these skills/processes helps you understand problems better and therefore allows you select the best strategy for solving them – a process you no doubt already carry out automatically.

The following example shows the different stages of problem solving:

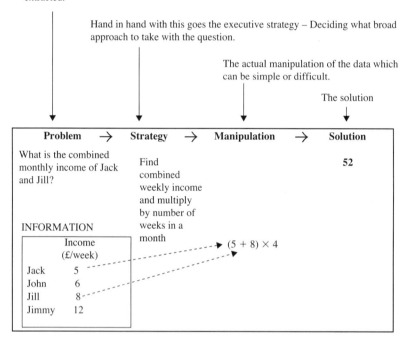

Part B: The approach

Numeracy

Number is a way of quantifying or measuring how big or how much something is. Numbers can best be thought of as being on a continuous line or "continuum" starting at zero. Numeracy involves manipulating numbers by means of numerical functions.

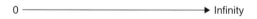

0 ⟶ Infinity

Basic function areas

Simple functions

"Simple" functions are one of the following four basic numerical functions:

● Addition
● Subtraction

- Multiplication
- Division.

Obviously you will be very familiar with these functions and how to use them. Everyone knows *how* to add, subtract, divide and multiply but what do these functions actually mean? Let us take a brief look at them.

Consider the *number line* above. Think about these functions in the context of changes on a number line. Addition is moving forward along the number line. Subtraction is moving backward/down along it; alternatively it can be thought of as the "gap" between two numbers on the line, and this is often an easier approach when more difficult subtractions are involved.

Take for example the sum **935 − 537**.

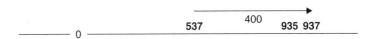

When thinking about the difference between numbers it is often easier to ask yourself: "what is the gap between them?" or "what do I need to add to the lower number to reach the higher number?" In this particular example, it is immediately obvious that adding 400 to 537 gives 937. The target of 935 is only 2 less than this; therefore 400 − 2 (398) gives the answer.

Multiplication can be thought of as adding a number to itself many times over. Whereas when you divide by "*n*" you are effectively asking yourself, how large would each "piece" be if a line were divided into "*n*" equal parts?

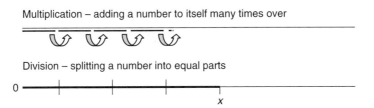

Multiplication – adding a number to itself many times over

Division – splitting a number into equal parts

These ideas are food for thought. It is not necessary to think deeply about these things when only simple numeracy problems are involved; but in complicated problems you may find it helpful to think what these processes actually entail.

Sums can be done in three main ways: in our head, on paper or on a calculator. Although we are generally calculator prone, the most effective method is a combination of mental arithmetic with the aid of pen and paper. Mental arithmetic can actually be a very powerful tool and can be quicker than either of the other options alone on occasions. (Note that in the UKCAT, the calculator is an on-screen one that may be quite slow and frustrating to use and that in the BMAT you will not be allowed to use a calculator at all!)

Have a look at the following example:

For the following questions, use the data in the table below.

Job	Estimated		Actual	
	Time (hours)	Cost (£)	Time (hours)	Cost (£)
Wardrobe	16	350	32	120
Garage Door	15	300	20	200
Leaking Tap	0.5	5	0.5	2
Radiator	3	25	2	15
TV Aerial	2	55	2.5	50
Insulation	10	200	8	150

Problem: *What was the total time taken to complete all the jobs?*

Strategy: add the values for "actual" time
Solution: $32 + 20 + 0.5 + 2 + 2.5 + 8 = 65$ hours

Problem: *What was the difference between estimated and actual total cost?*

Strategy: Total actual cost − Total estimated cost
Solution: $(120 + 200 + 2 + 15 + 50 + 150)$
$$- (350 + 300 + 5 + 25 + 55 + 200) = 537 - 935$$
$$= £398$$

When calculating "in your head", there is an easy way or path of least resistance to carry out any set of functions. For adding up strings of numbers, for instance, it is always easier to break it up into components that give you "easy numbers".

Easy numbers: These are numbers with which it is quick and easy to carry out functions. When you have a string of numbers, grouping these into "easy" numbers make other functions easier.
For example, the sum:
$$32 + 20 + 0.5 + 2 + 2.5 + 8$$
can be more easily tackled mentally as follows:
$$(32 + 20) + (2 + 8) + (2.5 + 0.5).$$

Problem: *What is the hourly cost of fixing the TV aerial?*

Strategy: Divide total cost by hours worked
Solution: 50/2.5 = £20/hour

Problem: *How much time would it take to fix 6 wardrobes (using "Estimated" figures)?*

Strategy: Multiply estimated time per wardrobe by 6.
Solution: $6 \times 16 = (6 \times 10) + (6 \times 6) = 60 + 36 = 96$

You are provided with number drills at various points in this chapter. Make sure to time yourself and feel free to review them as many times as you wish, noting how your speed changes.

Quick test 1

Number drill
(Calculator not allowed!)

1 (30 + 60 + 180)/1000
2 (5 + 4 + 3 + 2 + 1) × 4
3 33 + 16 + 12 + 89 + 145
4 1036 − (12 + 48 + 156)
5 589 × 42
6 349,239/16,899 (nearest whole number)
7 500/36 (nearest whole number)
8 36/5 (nearest decimal place)
9 2/200 − 2/50 (nearest decimal place)
10 1/(0.75 × 0.8) (as a whole number fraction)

Percentages/Ratios/Fractions
Percentages, ratios and fractions all do the same thing: they compare one number with another.
    The following illustration demonstrates this:

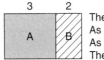

The absolute value of 'A' is 3
As a fraction of the total A = 3/5
As a percentage of the total A = 60% (60/100)
The ratio of A:B is 3:2

Another way to think about a fraction or percentage is as a part of a whole, with the "part" expressed by the *numerator* and the "whole" expressed by the *denominator*. As long as the fraction remains the same, the relationship between them must always be constant therefore any change to one must be reflected in the other. (A the denominator or "whole" is always 100.)

The following graph shows sales for different models of a car.

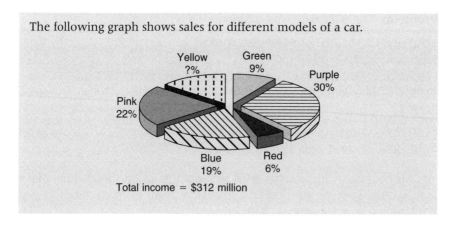

Total income = $312 million

Problem: *What was the income from yellow cars?*

Strategy: Here, as in any percentage problem, the "whole" pie chart is equal to 100, therefore the missing "piece" is simply 100 minus all the other parts.
Solution: $100 - 9 - 30 - 6 - 19 - 22 = 14\%$
So income from yellow cars is 14% of the total, or:

$$(14/100) \times \$312 \text{ million} = \$43,680,000$$

Problem: *What percentage of the total does an income of $12 million represent?*

Strategy: The total income (denominator) is 312 million, so we need to find the equivalent percentage representing the fraction 12/312 . . .
Solution:

$$\frac{12}{312} = \frac{x}{100} \rightarrow x = 100 \times \frac{12}{312} = 3.85\%$$

Problem: *If next year the income from green cars is $25 million and the income fraction from green cars remains the same, what will be the new total income?*

Strategy: We already know the income *fraction* for green cars is 9% (or 9/100). Next year, we are told this fraction amounts to $25 million. So:
Solution:

$$\frac{\$25 \text{ million}}{\text{Total income}} = 9\%$$

$$\$25,000,000 = \frac{9}{100} \times \text{total income}$$

$$\text{So total income} = \frac{\$2,500,000,000}{9} = \$277,777,777$$

Problem: *What is the ratio of the number of Red: Green: Purple cars sold?*

Strategy: Whereas the fraction compares one part to the whole, the ratio compares one part to another part.

The question asks us about the actual *number* sold – the number sold would be the total sales from each type of car divided by the cost *per car*. In this case, although the ratio of *sales* of red: green: purple would be 6:9:30 (or 2:3:10), the ratio of the *number* of cars would be:

$$\frac{6}{\text{Price of red car}} : \frac{9}{\text{Price of green car}} : \frac{30}{\text{Price of purple car}}$$

Since we don't know the price of each type of car, we cannot go any further.

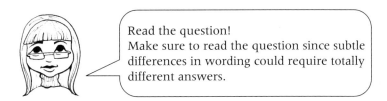

Read the question!
Make sure to read the question since subtle differences in wording could require totally different answers.

Another important and common type of function is *percentage change*. When we calculate a percentage change we are doing two things:

1 Calculating the actual or absolute change (i.e. a subtraction).
2 Expressing that difference as a percentage of the *original* amount.

Again, it can be useful to think about this in terms of the number line:

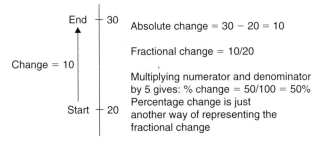

End ── 30   Absolute change = 30 − 20 = 10

Fractional change = 10/20

Change = 10   Multiplying numerator and denominator by 5 gives: % change = 50/100 = 50%
Percentage change is just
Start ── 20   another way of representing the fractional change

Working out the percentage change is often not too difficult. But it is very useful to remember this concept when it comes to working "backwards".
Take the following example:

Viewing figures for terrestrial TV last year were 24,450,362 (a 13% reduction from the previous year). What were the figures in the previous year?

Start
(Previous year) | x

1. Intuitive approach
Last year's figures were a 13% reduction from the previous year, that is a reduction of 13 for every 100. So if the previous year's figures was x, last years figures must be 87% (100−13) of x, so.

$$0.87x = 24,450,362$$
$$x = 28,103,864$$

Change
(13%)

2. Arithmetic/algebraic approach
Percentage change = 13% = 13/100

Fractional change = $\dfrac{x - 24,450,362}{x}$

End
(Last Year) | 24,450,362

$$\frac{(x - 24,450,362)}{x} = \frac{13}{100}$$

$$x - 24,450,362 = 0.13x$$

$$0.87x = 24,450,362$$

Note that the answer is *not* 13% of 24,450,362 added to it, Therefore x = 28,103,864 (a common mistake) since 24,450,362 is not the start value but the end product of the percentage change.

Percentage change
- *Always make sure you are certain about the "start" and "end" points of any percentage change.*
- Understand that fractions and percentages do not exist on their own; they always refer to something – *a baseline value* or *Start point*. A percentage change occurs when you take a fraction of a *certain baseline value* and add it to or remove it from that same value.
- 120 is 20% greater than *100* but 96 (not 100) is 20% smaller than *120*. The first 20% is as a fraction of 100 but the second 20% is as a fraction of 120.

Quick test 2

For the following questions, use the data in the table below:

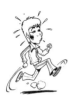

	Sales (000s £)
1994	400
1995	385
1996	?
1997	542
1998	650

1 What is the percentage change in sales from 1994 to 1995?
2 If sales were projected to increase by 2% from 1994 to 1995, what is the shortfall in sales in 1995, compared with projected figures?
3 Bob calculates that the figures for 1998 are 20% higher than the previous year. Is Bob correct?

4 The figure for 1997 represents a 12.5% increase from the previous year. Fill in the figure for 1996.

5 The percentage change in sales is projected to be 10% higher from last year to this year than between 1996 and 1997. If sales were £1,320,000 last year, what is the value of predicted sales this year?

Quick test 3

The graph shows the change in bonus payments of different employees from last year, including Bob (represented by a square) and Bill (represented by a circle).

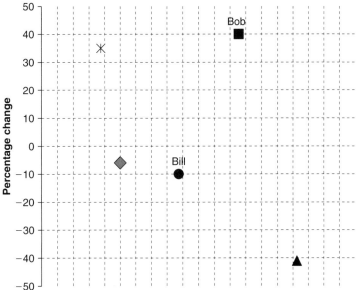

1 If last year Bob and Bill both earned a fixed income of £120,000 and bonuses of £10,000 and £15,000, respectively, what is the difference between their incomes this year?

2 If last year Bob and Bill both earned a fixed income of £120,000 and bonuses of 10,000 and 15,000, respectively, by what percentage does Bills Fixed income have to increase this year in order for his take-home pay to exceed Bob's? (Assume Bob's fixed income remains the same).

3 A 6th employee, Brad's bonus is not represented in the above graph. By what percentage would his bonus payment had to have changed so that the average percentage change in bonus is not affected?

Specific (Applied) Functions
Time
Most of us are familiar with the way time is measured, learning to tell the time and date as early as primary school. But like most functions covered

in this chapter we don't often give the concept of time, clocks and calendars more than rudimentary thought. This part of the chapter hopes to give you the opportunity to *think* a little more about this function.

Quick test 4

Number drill

(No calculator!)

How many seconds in 1 day?
How many minutes in a week?
How many hours in January?

The analogue clock measures the hours of the day using numbers 1–12 while the 24-hour clock uses numbers 0–23.

> The 14:43 train actually arrives at the platform at 8 p.m. and further delays of 42 minutes occur before it departs. What is the total delay to the start of the journey?

Firstly calculate the time that has elapsed from 14:43 to 20:00:

$$20:00 - 14:43 = 05:17.$$

Secondly add the further delay of 42 minutes:

$$05:17 + 42 = 05:59$$

Answer: 5 hours 59 minutes delay.

Subtraction of times can be thought of in just the same way as conventional numbers – think of a "time line" instead of the number line.

> I wake up in the middle of the night: my digital clock reads 23:43. I am woken up again at 06:30 by my alarm clock. How many complete circles did the minute hand of my analogue watch make between these two times?

Think about the position of the analogue watch at the time I was woken (i.e. at 11:43 p.m.). For each complete circle, the minute hand would have to move all the way around to 43 minutes past the hour.

Complete circles	Time
1	00:43
2	01:43
3	02:43
4	03:43
5	04:43
6	05:43

The next time it makes a full circle it will be 6:43 but I wake up at 06:30, so answer is *six times*.

It is 3 p.m. By 3:20 p.m., how far will the hour hand have moved?

1HR=60 M
20

Think about how the hour hand and minute hand move in relation to one another. Using this example, the hour hand would move from 3 to 4 when the minute hand moves all the way around the face of the clock (i.e. from 12 to 12).

In other words the hour hand moves the equivalent of 5 "minutes" every time the minute hand moves 60 minutes. Therefore in 20 minutes the hour hand would move a third of the distance between 3 and 4 p.m. (20/60 = 1/3).

$$\frac{\text{No. of minutes moved by hour hand}}{\text{No. of minutes moved by minute hand}} = \frac{5}{60}$$

What is the angle between the hour and minute hands of the clock when it is 9:00?

The angle round a clock, like any circle, is 360°.

If you know what fraction of the circumference the angle subtends then you can calculate what fraction of 360 the angle is.

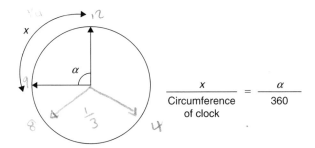

$$\frac{x}{\text{Circumference of clock}} = \frac{\alpha}{360}$$

At 9:00. The hour hand is on 9 and the minute hand is on 12.
So the distance between them is ¼ of the circumference of the clock.

So the angle between them is ¼ × 360° = 90°.

> What is the angle between the hour and minute hands of the clock when it is 8:20?

The same principle applies to this question.

You might think that because at 8:20 the hour hand is on 8 and the minute hand is on 4 then you might calculate the angle as $(8 - 4)/12 \times 360 = 120°$.

But this would be wrong because at 8:20 the hour hand is not on 8 but is somewhere between 8 and 9. So we must first find out where exactly it is and then calculate the angle.

At 8 the hour hand was on 8, since then the minute hand has moved 20 minutes. Using our understanding of ratios:

$$\frac{20 \text{ minutes}}{\text{Minutes moved by hour hand}} = \frac{60}{5}$$

So minutes moved by hour hand is $100/60 = 1.66$ minutes.

So the hour hand is about 1.66 "minutes" from 8 on the clock.

So the angle between them = $20 + 1.66 = 21.66/60 \times 360° = 129.96°$.

Quick test 5

1 If the 4:56 train will be approximately 4 hours 13 minutes late at what time will it arrive?
2 How long has it taken me to travel from London to New York, if my time of departure was 8:43 a.m. (London time) and my time of arrival was 3:32 p.m. (New York time) and if New York is 5 hours behind London?
3 The clock shows the time as being 3:45. If, by 4 p.m. the minute hand has covered a circumference of 18 cm, what distance has the hour hand covered?
4 What is the angle between the minute and hour hands of the clock when it is 8:24?

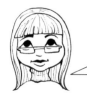

1 To improve your speed at doing time-calculations:
(a) Think of the "time line"
(b) Practice! (mental arithmetic involving times).
2 Think about the relationship between analogue and digital time; and in analogue time the relation between the hour and minute hands.

Calendar

There are just a few things to bear in mind with calculations involving calendars.

Firstly, different months have different days – 28, 29, 30 or 31 depending on the month – (use this information in calculations if you know which months are involved!).

Secondly, common approximations that we use in day-to-day life (such as, "4 weeks in a month", "30 days in a month") are not always safe to use in calculations.

If there are roughly 4 weeks in a month and 12 months in a year, that means there must be 48 weeks in a year. True or False? *Why?*

What is a leap year? Why do we have them?

The following shows the page of a calendar from February and early March in a particular year.

MON	TUE	WED	THU	FRI	SAT	SUN
			1	2	3	4
5	6	7	8	9	10	11
12	13	14	15	16	17	18
19	20	21	22	23	24	<u>25</u>
26	27	28	1	2	3	<u>4</u>

In *this* year, John and Jack both have birthdays that fall on Sundays (on 25th February and 4th March, respectively).

1 After Jack's birthday how many weeks will elapse before a Sunday falls on a date which is a multiple of 4?

2 If next year is a leap year, on what days of the week will their birthdays fall?

3 If next year is a leap year, how many days before their birthdays both fall on a Sunday again?

1 Counting the dates over months which are comprised of different numbers of days can be a bit tricky. It can help to use a pictorial representation for example like the following diagram:

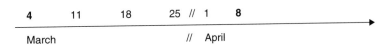

4   11   18   25 // 1   8

March   // April

Here we have jotted down the dates of all the subsequent Sundays (being mindful of the total number of days in each month). From this it is clear that this will next happen 5 weeks later on 8th April.

2 Each year, the day of the week on which a given date falls shifts along by one day; e.g. if this year, 29th June is a Monday, next year it will be a Tuesday. The significance of the leap year is that the additional day at the end of February shifts this by one extra day for every date after it.

   If it was not a leap year, both birthdays would fall on Mondays next year. However, in a leap year, Jack's birthday (25th February), which lies before the added day at 29th February will be on a Monday, however this added day will cause John's birthday (4th March) to be not on a Monday but on a Tuesday.

3 First we should try and find when one of the birthdays (let's take 25th February) next falls on the same day. This is best figured out using a diagram to help visualise things. Let's say this year is 2007 and next year is 2008 (leap year), we can fill in which days the 25th February falls on in each year subsequently.

MON	TUE	WED	THU	FRI	SAT	SUN
						2007
2008		2009	2010	2011	**2012**	
2013	2014	2015	**2016**		2017	**2018**

Leap years

(Note that after every leap year, there is a "jump" of two days for earlier dates.)

   From this we can see that the 25th February will next fall on a Sunday in 2018. Jack's birthday (4th March) should also fall on a Sunday on this year as it is not a leap year. There are 11 years (3 leap years) therefore:

   $(11 \times 365) + 3 = 4018$ days during this period.

Quick test 6

1 If March 1st is a Sunday, how many Sundays are there in March?

2 The year is 1994. It is Sunday and it is the 18th of December. When next will the same date in a month be a Sunday?

3 A man makes a mistake when filling out a form. He was meant to enter his birth date in the form DD:MM:YY but instead entered the time from his digital watch (a 24-hour clock, showing hours, minutes and seconds). The error was not detected early because the entry was plausible (i.e. it could have truly been his birth date). Which one of the following could possibly be his date of birth? (In each case if not, state why not.)

A 12th January 1984
B 15th December 1938
C 1st March 1960
D 28th June 1900

Questions 4 to 6 refer to the following information:
The year is 1982. Jim underlines his birthday on his calendar (below)

December						
MON	**TUE**	**WED**	**THU**	**FRI**	**SAT**	**SUN**
		1	2	3	4	5
6	7	8	9	10	11	12
13	14	<u>15</u>	16	17	18	19
20	21	22	23	24	25	26
27	28	29	30	31		

4 On what day of the week will his next birthday fall?
5 How many Sundays will fall between the New Year (1983) and Jim's next birthday?
6 Next year (1983) how many months will have three or more even-dated Wednesdays?

Money
Use of money is common and essential to everyday life. We also convert money from one currency to another. Calculations involving money are probably the most common numerical activity performed by the general public. Therefore being confident dealing with numbers in the form of money is very useful. Money-related problems also bring in many other numerical skills. When money is converted from one currency to the other, this brings in the topic of ratios and fractions.

Quick test 7

Number drill
Calculate the following (not using a calculator!):

1 (£4.52 + £3.88 + £12.67) ×12
2 12% of £3.85
3 A 30% increase on your answer to question 1
4 What is the percentage profit made by a shopkeeper who sells 12 vases at £34.99 per vase, each costing him £24.99?
5 If £2 buys me $3.80, how much will a $550.00 airplane ticket cost in pounds?

In every country, there is a system of organising money into different "denominations" or discrete values. This system, like any other, has rules – therefore another potential territory for specifically testing problem-solving skills!

The Monetary System: example using pounds and pence

100p = £1
Notes: £5, £10, £20, £50
Coins: 1p, 2p, 5p, 10p, 20p, 50p, £1, £2

I want to buy a shirt with a price of £41 and I only have a £50 note. The cashier has only 20 coins (consisting of 50p and 20p coins only). After the transaction what combination of notes and coins would allow me to have the maximum number of 20p coins (and still receive exact change)?

Firstly, breakdown the question (which is quite "wordy") and ask yourself, *what* do I need to find out? In this case, the change is £9.00 exactly.

Therefore the problem is how do I make £9.00 change using notes and 20ps and 50ps (up to a maximum of 20 in total), so that the *number of 20p coins* is maximised?

Strategy: The strategy to maximise the coins is to use as many 20p coins as possible and as few 50p coins as possible (within the rules we have been told).

Solution:

- *Set the limits*: We don't know the exact number of each type of coin but the cashier clearly has at least 1 of each type, so the maximum number of either type of coin he could have is 19.
- We could make the full amount using 18 × 50p's (= £9.00), but obviously this would not give us any 20p coins.
- If he gave us 19 × 20p coins, we would have £3.80 (this cannot be made up to a whole number using 50p coins alone).
- By now you can see that we will need to use a £5 note and try and make £4.00 with the coins.
- The next number of 20p coins he could give us and still make it up to £4.00 is 15 (15 × 20p = £3.00).
- Therefore the answer is *(15 × 20p's) + (2 × 50p's) + £5 note*.

Quick test 8

1 How many "amounts" of money between £5 and £10 can be made up using an equal number of notes and coins?

The graph below shows the total value of money in John's pocket over time.

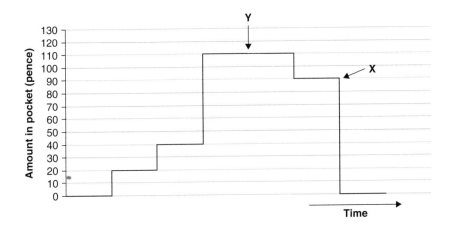

2 Based on the graph, what is/are
   (a) the minimum number
   (b) the maximum number
   of denomination(s) of coins he could have in his pocket throughout the
   time shown? Name them. (By denominations we mean the type of coin;
   e.g. 10p, 20p, 50p are three different "denominations".)
3 If at X, John took out a 50p piece from the same pocket, what are the
   minimum number of denominations he can have at Y?

The table below shows average exchange rates for converting pounds into
different currencies over a 6-month period (the figures in each cell show
how much of each currency can be bought with £1.00).

	January	February	March	April	May	June
£ → $	2.05	1.98	2.04	2.25	2.38	2.59
£ → Rs.	81	78	84	85	89	95
£ → Yuan	15.67	15.71	15.69	15.66	15.63	15.68

4 How much would a Rs. 14.00 item cost in pounds (£)?
5 What is the percentage change in the value of the dollar ($) between
   April and June?
6 How many Dollars could one buy with 1000 Yuan in April?
7 What is the profit margin one would make over the 6 months by buing
   Yuan instead of Dollars in January (express your answer as a percentage).

Shapes

A look at 2D and 3D functions
Lines: These are the basic components of shapes.
Perimeter: The distance around a shape is called the perimeter. It is a linear
measurement, i.e. it just involves measuring a line.

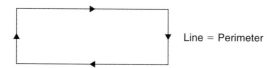

Line = Perimeter

Area: When you have one or more lines meet up to form a closed off area you have a regular shape. It is a square measurement (x^2) because it involves multiplying 2 lines (linear parameters). These kinds of shapes will be referred to as 2-dimensional (2D) objects.

Some common shapes

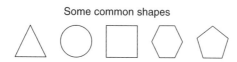

Concept of Area: This horizontal line multiplied by the length of this vertical line give the measurement of area:

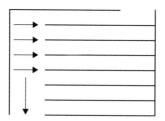

Volume: If you stack many "areas" one on top of another, you get a volume. "Real" objects (i.e. objects you can actually hold) have volume. It involves three linear parameters (the length, breath and thickness of the stack). These objects are referred to as 3D objects.

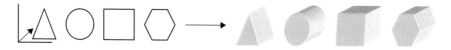

Quick test 9

1 What are the areas of common shapes (i.e. triangle, circle, square, etc.)?
2 What are the volumes of common solids?

Although it is important to understand area and volume, a Thinking Skills test such as the BMAT is unlikely to test this understanding directly. Instead you are usually required to perform some *manipulation* of spatial information.

This is the same principle as all the previous functions already discussed in this chapter but the information presented in this case is spatial.

Folding

Now that we understand the basics of shapes and objects generally, an important problem-solving skill is to be able to fold 2D shapes. The way a shape looks when it is folded depends on the lines along which it is folded. An object can be folded along any line you choose but if it is to be folded in half it must be folded along a line of symmetry.

Take this circle, for example. It has two small bits missing at opposite ends. Imagine we are asked to fold it in half twice; there are several possible outcomes. These of course depend on the lines along which it is folded. What each diagram shows is the result when it is folded twice along the lines of symmetry shown.

If we fold it along the dotted lines shown in Diagram A, it will look like Ai from both sides. If we fold it along the lines shown in Diagram B, it may look like Bi or Bii depending on which side we look at.

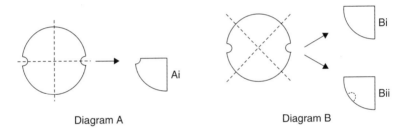

Diagram A   Diagram B

Quick test 10

1 You are presented with three different hexagonal shapes – A, B and C, with different parts carved out. Each of them is folded in half, first once and then twice.

   Can you match each of the folded objects with one or more of the original shapes?

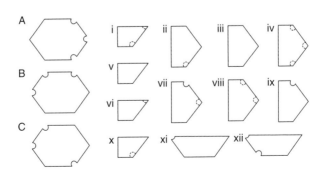

Rotations and Reflections

Rotations

Another manipulative skill is the ability to rotate 3D objects and thus determine how they might look from different angles. Below are different sets of 3D objects which have been rotated to give different views. Try to determine which views are possible and which are not and why.

Are these two possible views of the same object?

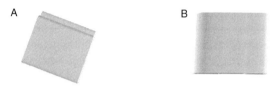

Yes they are. We are shown end-on views in both cases, so it is possible that they are end-on views of different sides of the same object. You must be careful here as we cannot be certain that they are exactly the same object. But it is *possible* that they are.

Are these two possible views of the same object?

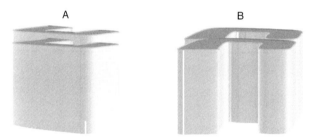

No, they are not. In A, the two horse-shoe parts of the shape are not as aligned in the same way as B. We are able to tell this because we are given more than just an end-on view.

Quick test 11

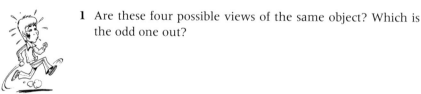

1 Are these four possible views of the same object? Which is the odd one out?

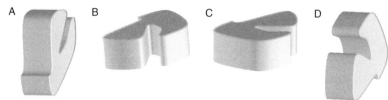

2 Are these two possible views of the same object?

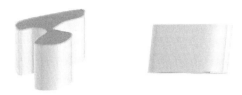

Reflections

Understanding the way mirrors work is fundamental but can be quite tricky. As shown in the diagram below a mirror performs *lateral inversion*. What this means is that each equivalent point on the *object* and in the *image* is the same distance from the mirror and directly opposite each other.

In this first example point 1 on the object is the same distance from point 1 on the image and they are directly opposite each other (i.e. the line attaching them is perpendicular to the mirror). This is the same for points 2, 3, 4, and 5.

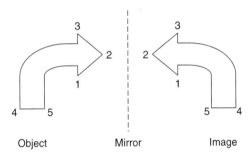

In the next example, point A on the object and point A on the image are directly opposite each other and are equidistant from the mirror. Also consider how the curves are reflected; a curve to the right becomes a curve to the left when reflected and a curve to the left becomes a curve to the right when reflected.

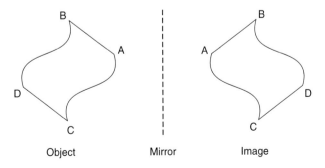

Quick test 12

1 Based on the reflection principle and using a ruler can you draw the correct images of the following objects in the mirror.

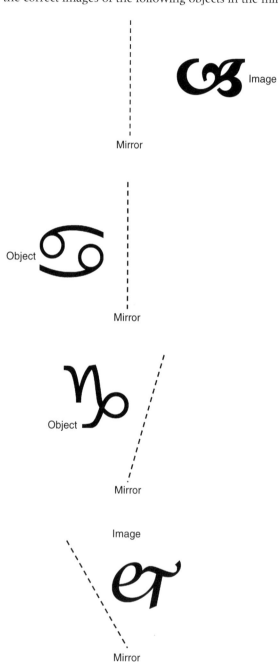

2D to 3D conversion

It is also important to be able to convert 2D objects to 3D objects or at least imagine the 2D views of 3D objects. 2D–3D conversion is very important as in "real life" we often represent 3D objects as plain 2D drawings and it is important to be able to deduce important information like proportions and relative positions from this limited information.

Below is a 3D object. Which of the following (A to D) is a possible view of one of the sides of the object?

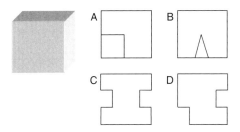

In this example, we are shown 3 sides of a cube, 9 edges, partial views of 6 corners and a full view of 1 corner. There could be a lot going on in the edges, corners and sides hidden from view so we must be imaginative.

Option A is possible as there could be a square-shaped chunk missing from the corner out of our view.

Option B is also possible as there could be a triangular chunk missing from one of the edges out of our view.

Option C is *not* possible as there are two long chunks missing on opposite sides. We would be aware of this as we can see half of the sides of the cube.

Option D is also *not* possible for the same reason as option C.

Quick test 13

1 Figure X is a side on view of an object. Which of the options (A to D) is a possible top view of the same object (i.e. looking in the direction of the arrow).

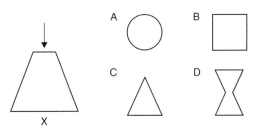

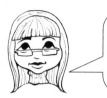

The key to spatial reasoning is familiarity which comes with practice. Why don't you take matters into your own hand: observe how everyday objects can be manipulated, how they look from different directions and how they look when reflected in a mirror.

Graphs

A graph or table is just another way of representing data. Although graphs are meant to be easily digestible forms of data representation, their interpretation can often be confusing so they are worth a separate look. There are different types of graphs which can be used in many different ways, depending on the emphasis required. Below are a few examples.

Bar graph

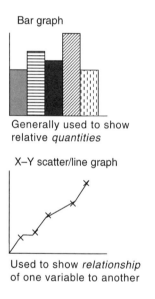

Generally used to show relative *quantities*

X–Y scatter/line graph

Used to show *relationship* of one variable to another

Pie chart

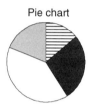

Used to show *fractions* of various components as part of the whole

There are several skills involved. These will test your ability to:

- Extract data
- Analyse the data in order to solve a problem
- Make inferences from the information
- Relate one graph or chart to another or a non-graphical form of data representation

Extracting and analysing data

The ability to extract and derive information from the graph is the most common and basic function you can do. It is extremely important to get a good grasp of what exactly the graph shows and, just as importantly, what it does *not* show. The first way to do this is by carefully looking at the axes or other parameters of the graphs and making sure you know exactly what each result or value means.

You may be asked to obtain two main types of information from a graph: (a) where the information is directly demonstrated; (b) where the information is not immediately obvious – for this latter type of question you have to ask yourself, "can this be derived from the information in the graph?"

The following graph shows the changes in average monthly temperature from one month to the next, during two separate winters, 2001–2002 and 2004–2005.

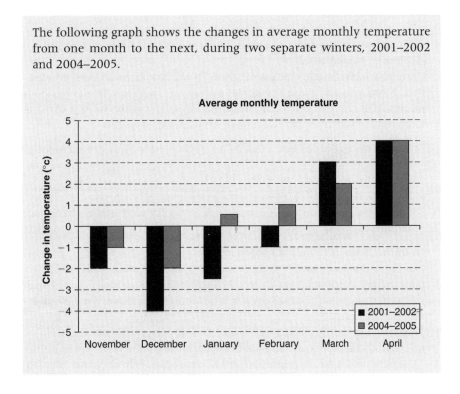

1 *What was the change in average monthly temperature from October 2001 to November 2001?*
Here you are asked to read directly from the graph. First ask yourself, "What does the graph show?" Each bar shows the change in average temperature from the previous month. The bar for November shows a temperature change of −2°C, therefore this is the answer.

2 *Which month was colder on average – April 2002 or April 2005?*
Here you are asked for something that is not directly evident from the graph. To answer this question, you need to know the *actual* temperature in each of these months. In this case the graph does *not* show actual

temperatures, only *change* in temperature; therefore you cannot tell which month was colder without further information.

3 *If the temperature on 28th November 2004 was 2°C, what was the temperature likely to be one month later?*
The answer is simply $2 - 4 = -2$°C, correct? Wrong! Look carefully again at the question. Ask yourself, "What do I need to know to answer this question?" – it asks for the temperature on a specific date based on the temperature on another single specific date. The information in the graph is based only on the average temperature for each month.

4 *If the average temperature in October 2001 was 14°C what was the average temperature in January 2002?*
Here you have to use the information in the graph to process information. Since you are given the actual average temperature in the previous month, you can use it with the information in the graph to calculate the temperature in November, December and January as follows:

Temperature in November 2001 $= 14 - 2 = 12$ (-2 is the change for November).
Temperature in December 2001 $= 12 - 4 = 8$ (-4 is the change for December).
Temperature in January 2002 $= 8 - 2.5 = 5.5$ (-2.5 is the change for January).

(A quicker way is to do it all together: $14 - 2 - 4 - 2.5 = 5.5$)

5 *If the average temperature in October 2001 and 2004 were the same, which Winter was colder on average? (Take Winter to mean the period between November–February inclusive.)*
This question can be done two ways:
(a) Give the temperature in October an arbitrary value and work out the temperature for each month from November to February and calculate the average for each year.
(b) Looking at the graph you can see that in the period between November and February the change in temperature for 2001–2002 is always lower (more negative) than that for 2004–2005, therefore you can conclude that the temperatures in every month in 2001–2002 will be colder if they are both starting at the same level and therefore the Winter of 2001–2002 as a whole will of course be colder on average.
(This strategy of "eye-balling" the graph for your answer is obviously much quicker than the first, but be warned, only use it if the difference is quite obvious.)

6 *Which 6-month period (November–April) was more variable in actual average temperature changes from month to month?*

Without going into formal statistical concepts such as "variance" etc. (which you would not be expected to know), we all know that the concept of variability is about the *degree of change* (irrespective of the direction, positive or negative). In this case, therefore, the one way to get an idea of this would be to add up the size of the bars for each group.

For 2001–2002, it is: 2 + 4 + 2.5 + 1 + 3 + 4 = 16.5
For 2004–2005, it is: 3 + 2 + 0.5 + 1 + 2 + 4 = 12.5

This gives us a general idea of degree of change or variability (although it is not a formal mathematical formula). Another way to see this difference is again by simply "eye-balling" the graph, where it is quite clear that the bars for 2001–2002 are larger.

With any graphical question ask yourself:
1 What does it show? (look at the axes!)
2 What does it **not** show?
Before looking back at the graph, ask yourself,
"What information do I need to answer this question?
   Does the graph show this information directly? If not, can it be derived from the graph with the information provided?"

The following is a cumulative frequency graph of the heights of 7-year-old children in a classroom in the town of Haverhurst.

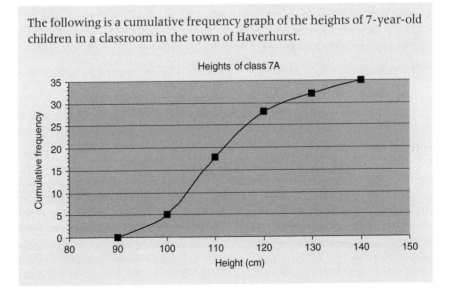

Heights of class 7A

1 *What is the height of the smallest pupil?*
What does the graph show? In this case the cumulative frequency at any height shows the number of pupils who are at that height *or lower*. (An even better way to imagine this is to think about how the graph was made: imagine if someone took a bar and placed it at 90 cm above the ground and then counted how many pupils came under it, and then repeated this for 100 cm, 110 cm, and so on. This is a good way to understand what cumulative frequency represents.) In this case we know that no pupils are 90 cm or lower, but 5 are 100 cm or lower (the smallest pupil is clearly somewhere in this group but his/her height maybe anything from 90.0000001 cm to 100 cm, according to the graph!), so we cannot tell what his actual height is.

2 *What is the mean height of the class?*
What do you need to calculate this? You need the height of each individual pupil which you add together and divide by the total number of pupils. The total number is easy – that's simply where the graph ends, i.e. 35. What about individual heights? Do you have this information? No. Can you derive it from the graph? No. Therefore the question cannot be answered.

3 *How many pupils are taller than 120 cm?*
What do you need to calculate this? Well, we know 28 students are 120 cm or lower. The rest, $(35 - 28) = 7$, must therefore be taller than this.

4 *How many pupils are between 100 cm and (up to and including) 120 cm tall?*
28 pupils are 120 cm or shorter
5 pupils are 100 cm or shorter

Therefore, $28 - 5 = 23$ pupils must lie in between. (In other words take away those pupils who are 100 cm or shorter from those who are 120 cm or shorter – think about the "bar" analogy described above.)

Inference
Inference is something you deduce from the graph without it directly being shown. This tests your understanding of the *implications* of the information presented and to deduce what this might mean when applied to different circumstances. It requires a certain amount of critical thinking about the information you derive from the graph.

Taking our previous examples, think about what you can and cannot infer or deduce from this information.

The following is a cumulative frequency graph of the heights of 7-year-old children in a classroom in the town of Haverhurst.

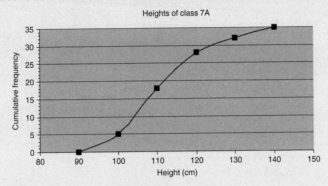

Heights of class 7A

Assuming that the average height of a 7-year-old nationally is 120 cm and that most children who are malnourished are shorter than average, which of the following can be reliably inferred about the pupils in Class 7A?

A Most pupils in Class 7A are probably malnourished
B Most pupils of Class 7A are shorter than average
C Less than a quarter of pupils in Class 7A are taller than average
D Generally, the pupils in Class 7A are less athletic than average
E Most pupils in 7A will be shorter than average as adults

Here we are given a new piece of information and have to infer from that. If we look at 120 cm on the graph, it is obvious that the majority of pupils in Class 7A fall below this height. So, looking at the statements:

Option A: We are told most children who are malnourished are short, but the converse, i.e. that most children who are short are malnourished does not necessarily apply. So it *cannot* be reliably inferred.

Option B: Since most of the pupils' heights fall below 120 cm it would be fair to say that most people in Class 7A are below average in height. So it is *true*.

Option C: Here some more analysis is needed. We know 28 of 35 are less than or equal to 120 cm. Therefore 7/35 (20%) are taller than 120 cm. So it is *true*.

Option D: This is quite irrelevant – there is nothing in the question to associate athleticism with height. So it *cannot* be reliably inferred. (*Remember*: use *only* the information in the question!)

Option E: This may or may not be true; however, we have no information on how a child's height at age 7 predicts their height in later life. So this *cannot* be reliably inferred.

One interesting and very common point emerging from this is what we call correlation (an association between things) and causality. It is a common pitfall to mistake the two. Take the following example.

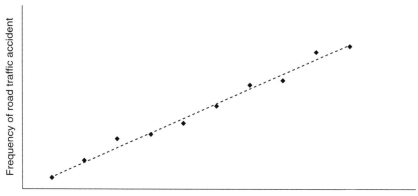

The graph shows a positive correlation (or association) between the likelihood of wearing jeans and having a road traffic accident. Does this mean that wearing jeans *causes* you or predisposes you to having an accident? Unlikely. There may be a common factor linking one thing to another (e.g. the younger you are the more likely you are to wear jeans and also the more likely you are to having an accident, due to inexperience at the wheel). Let us look at another example for inference.

The following graph shows the changes in average monthly temperature from one month to the next, during two separate winters, 2001–2002 and 2004–2005.

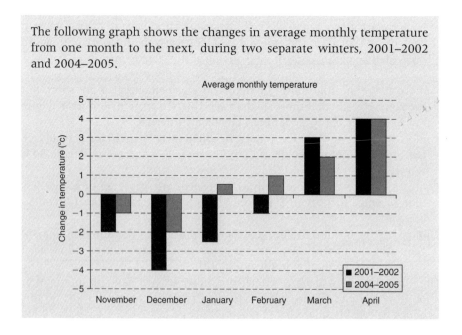

1 *If the average temperature in March is 12°C and the trend between March and April continues, what will be the average temperature in July 2005?*

The first thing to note here is that we cannot even begin answering this question if we are not told that the trend between March and April continues. Remember we cannot assume that because things have been going a certain way, they will continue going that way.

Next, we need to be careful to make sure what exactly is meant by "trend". Is it the absolute or relative trend?

The absolute trend is: +4°C from March to April therefore $(4 \times 4) = 16$°C from April to July, so the temperature in July will be 12°C + 16°C = 28°C. This is usually what is meant by such a question.

The relative trend looks at the change in temperature as a proportion of the original. In this case, the temperature in April is 16/12 (4/3) the temperature in March. If I sequentially multiply each result by 4/3 from month to month, I would get a very different answer. (Try it!)

Which number is next in the sequence: 100, 200, ...?
Is it 300 (200 + 100),
Or is it 400 (200 × 2)?

2 *Which of the following can be reliably inferred from the graph (assume that the average temperature in October 2001 and October 2004 were the same)?*
  A The Winter of 2006–2007 will be warmer than that of 2004–2005.
  B Since global warming causes warmer winters, this is clear evidence of global warming.
  C April 2005 was 6°C warmer than April 2002.
  D If the absolute difference in average monthly temperature between different years continues, the temperature in February 2002 would be 16°C warmer than in February 2008.

Let us go through each of these in turn

Option A: It is true that the winter of 2004–2005 is warmer. However it is *not* necessarily true that this trend will continue. So *cannot* be reliably inferred.

Option B: Although global warming may cause warmer winters, a warm winter is not necessarily caused by global warming (it may be caused by other things). So, *cannot* be reliably inferred.

Option C: We are told to assume that the temperature at the beginning of both winters is the same (let us call it "*x*"). If we simply add up the bars, the temperature in April 2005 would be $x + 4.5$; in April 2001 it would be $x - 2.5$, therefore the difference is 6°C. So it is *true*.

Option D: True. Assuming the same starting temperature, there is an 8°C difference in temperature between February 2002 and February 2005 (using the same method as above). This is equivalent to an 8/3 difference per year. Over 6 years (2002–2006) this would be a difference of 16°C (8/3×6). We are safe in using absolute trend as this is clearly stated in the question. So it is *true*.

The following graphs show data relating to house prices in the town of Bridgewater.

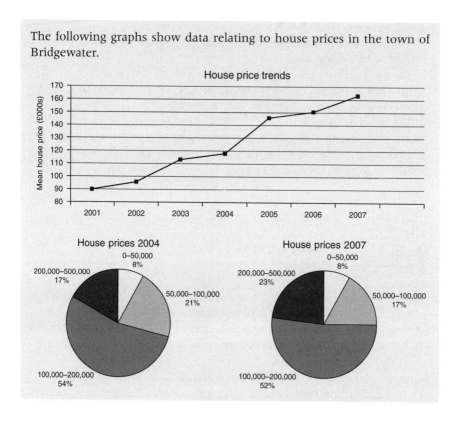

1 *What was the price of an average house in Bridgewater in 2004?*
£118,000 approximately (read off graph)

2 *What was the percentage difference in mean house prices between 2002 and 2004?*
Price in 2002 = £95,000
Price in 2004 = £118,000
Difference = 118,000 − 95,000 = 23,000
% Difference = (23,000/95,000) × 100 = 24%

3 *What was the difference between the actual house prices in 2007 compared with the house price predicted based on the absolute trend between 2002 and 2004?*
This question asks you to do 2 things:

1 Extrapolate the absolute trend between 2002 and 2004 to predict a price for 2007.
2 Compare that with the actual price for 2007.

The absolute difference between 2002 and 2004 is £23,000. This represents an increase of £11,500 per year. From 2002 to 2007 there are 5 years. Therefore if this trend continues the 2007 price would be (11,500 × 5) + 95,000 = £152,500.
The actual price in 2007 is £162,500 (from the graph).

Therefore the difference is £162,500 − £152,500 = £10,000

4 *Which of the following can be reliably inferred about house prices in Bridgewater?*
   A House prices will continue to increase.
   B Based on the absolute trend in the last 2 years, the average price in 2010 will be approximately £185,000.
   C The average house in 2006 would have to depreciate by approximately 40% to reach 2001 levels.
   D The acceleration in house price between 2004 and 2007 was caused by the increase in the proportion of £200,000–£500,000 houses.

Option A: Can't tell. There is no information to support this. (*Remember*: only use the information provided whatever your instinct or prior knowledge tells you!)
Option B: True. There is an approximately £8,000 per year increase between 2005 and 2007; therefore by 2010 this trend should reach approximately £185,000 when extrapolated.
Option C: True.
   2006 price = £150,000
   2001 price = £90,000
   Difference = £60,000
Percentage difference = 60/150 × 100 = 40%
   Note: "depreciation" is a change in the downward direction. It is treated exactly the same as any other change, but remembering that the "*starting point*" is the higher value (150,000) not the lower one (90,000), therefore we use this as the denominator.
Option D: False. It is true there was an acceleration in house price from 2004. From the pie chart we can see that there was also an increase in proportion of the £200,000–£500,000 houses. However, the pie chart simply reflects this increase in average house price in a different form. It does not tell us about underlying causes.

5 *Which of the following may explain the trend in house prices after 2004?*
   A General market forces such as reductions in interest rates making consumers more likely to buy a house.
   B Increase in local demand for homes.
   C A new development of luxury apartments at an average price of £350,000 each.
   D A relative increase in the number of £50,000–£100,000 homes between 2004 and 2007.

With this type of question the emphasis changes. The key word here is *"may"* – this should prompt you to now consider each possibility more generally and ask "could this possibly be a link?" Also notice that the question specifically refers to the trend after 2004; implicit in this question is the reference to the clear *change* in the trend after 2004 – as you can see the graph becomes steeper at this point.

Option A: True. A general entity such as this is almost always possibly a factor.

Option B: True. If demand increases, one can conceive prices increasing.

Option C: True. As you can see, this is well above the average house price and therefore may cause a steeper rise in average house price on top of the current trend; it also fits in the changes shown in the pie chart.

Option D: False. These houses are lower than average even at 2004. Therefore an increase in this bracket would tend to pull average prices down. Also, if you look at the pie chart you will see that the proportion of houses in this bracket actually decreases between these 2 years.

Relating graphs: Analogy

Finally you may be required to relate the information (or part of it) presented in one graphical form to that presented in another form. This involves spotting analogy or patterns between graphs.

The following table shows the finishing times for six different cyclists after a race.

Cyclist no.	X01	X12	A34	A51	BX2	GT5
Time	01:42	02:58	03:31	01:12	01:55	03:30

Which of the following graphs correctly represents this information?

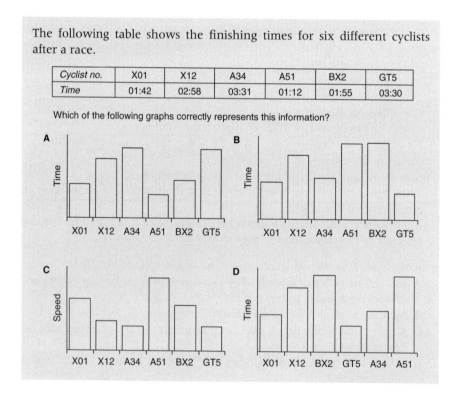

The general principle is that the numerical quantity is reflected by the size of the bar. Therefore, the relative sizes of the bars should reflect the times.

Graph A is correct since it correctly reflects the relative times of the different cyclists.

Graph B is wrong since it doesn't. The quick way to pick this up is to look for the obvious differences. For example it shows cyclists A51 and BX2 having the same times, but they clearly do not; also, it shows that GT5 has the quickest time, whereas he is actually one of the slowest.

Graph C is actually correct. The axis is *speed* not *time*. We know that speed is inversely proportional to time therefore the relative heights for speed should be exactly the opposite for time. Compare its shape with graph A.

Graph D seems to have exactly the same shape as A however, if you look carefully, the order of the cyclists is different. Therefore it doesn't accurately reflect the relative times of the cyclists.

Make sure you know what *each* graph represents separately, before drawing links between graphs.

The graph below shows how the incidence (or frequency) of respiratory diseases relates to the percentage of total medical consultations that are due to respiratory problems over a period of time.

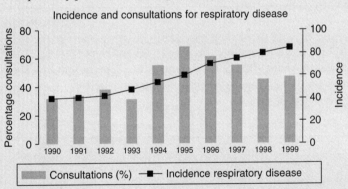

The Disease-Related Consultation Index (DRCI) looks at how the consultations for a particular disease as a proportion of all medical consultations changes with a change in the incidence of the disease from one year to the next, and is calculated as:

$$\frac{\text{Change in consultation rate}}{\text{Change in incidence of disease}}$$

Which of the following graphs could represent the change in DRCI for Respiratory disease over the period shown?

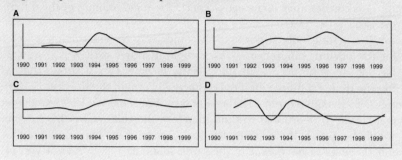

Here we are asked to consider the change in two variables in relation to one another. The best way to approach it is to take one at a time. Consider how the consultation rate changes from one year to the next (remember you are looking at the *change* between consecutive years, not the absolute trend). Now think how dividing each change by the change in incidence will alter it. To simplify this, concentrate on the major changes. Now look at the available options.

A Correct – this could be a change in the DRCI.
B Incorrect – this shows the change in incidence only.
C Incorrect – this reflects the absolute value of consultation rate.
D Also correct!

The following graph shows the speeds (in miles per hour) of the fastest (A) and slowest (B) cyclists during a race. The dotted line shows the average speed of all the cyclists during the same period.

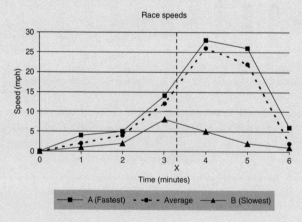

1 *Which of the following box plots best represents the distribution of speeds for all the cyclists at X?*

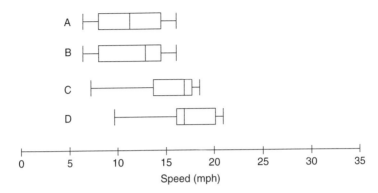

The answer is C because the maximum, minimum and mean values line up.

2 *How much further does A travel than B between 2 and 3 minutes?*
Average speed = Distance/time. Between 2 and 3 minutes, the speed of A increases at a constant rate from 5 to 15 mph; and B increases from 2 to 7 mph.

Average speed of A = speed at 2.5 minutes = 10 mph
Distance = speed × time = 10 mph × 1/60 hour = 0.1666 miles

Average speed B = speed at 2.5 minutes = 5 mph
Distance = speed × time = 5 mph × 1/60 hour = 0.0833 miles

Therefore difference in distance = 0.1666−0.0833 = 0.0833 miles

Another way to do this is to measure the area between both lines on the graph during this period as the area under the speed–time graph is a function of distance (speed × time).

3 *At 1 minute, how fast should B travel in order to catch up with A within the next minute?*
To catch up with A, B should reach the distance travelled by A at 2 minutes.
Therefore during the second minute B must travel:
Distance travelled by A at 2 minutes − Distance travelled by himself at 1 minute

Distance travelled by A at 2 minutes:
Distance travelled in first minute = average speed × time
                                     = 2 mph × 1/60 = 2/60
Distance travelled in 2nd minute = average speed × time
                                     = 4.5 mph × 1/60 = 4.5/60
                                     = 2/60 + 4.5/60 = 6.5/60

Distance travelled by B at 1 minute = Average speed × time
$$= 0.5\,\text{mph} \times 1/60 = 1/120$$
Distance for B to catch up between 1 and 2 minutes = 6.5/60 − 1/120
$$= 13/120 - 1/120 = 12/120 = 1/10\ \text{miles}$$

Since speed = Distance/time

Speed needed by B to catch up = (1/10)/(1/60) = 1/10 × 60 = 6 mph

4 *Which of the following best reflects the distance between A and B during the period of the graph?*

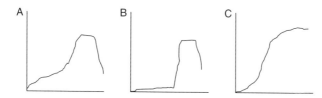

Think about this question carefully. Remember that the graph shows the relative *speeds* of the two cyclists. This means that whenever the speed of A is greater than B, he will be moving further and further away (that is his *distance* will be increasing). If this difference remains constant, the distance between them will *increase* at a constant rate. The slope of the distance graph reflects the difference in speed. If the relative speed increases, this slope will increase; if the difference in speed decreases (as towards the end of the graph) it will reduce. When B and A travel at the same speed, the gap between the vehicles stays constant and therefore the distance graph will flatten. Only when B's speed exceeds A's will the gap between them close and the distance graph slope downwards. From this fact alone you can see that only the third graph is correct. (The first copies the speed graph of A and the second shows the difference in speed between A and B.)

Broad themes: Combining functions

Rates

We have rates when one variable changes with change in tune with another variable. In other words one is dependent on the other. A very familiar example of a type of rate is speed. Speed is a common theme of problem-solving questions. Although knowing the formulae is mostly helpful, it can actually be intrusive and prevent you from approaching such questions intuitively. Let's take a look at speed and some other types of rate.

Speed and Flow Rates
Speed = Distance/time
Distance = Speed × time and time = Distance/speed.

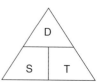

A car moves at 100 km/hour, how long before it covers a distance of (a) 100 km, (b) 200 km and (c) 250 km?

There are two ways to solve this.

1 Use the formula (time = distance/speed) in which case the answers are (a) 100/100 = 1 hour, (b) 200/100 = 2 hours and (c) 250/100 = 2.5 hours.
2 On the other hand you can think about the question intuitively. In which case since the car covers 100 km every hour (a) it will take 1 hour to cover 100 km, (b) it will take twice this time to cover 200 km = 2 hours and (c) 2.5 times as long to cover 250 km = 2.5 hours.

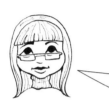

Thinking about things intuitively helps to solve difficult problems and can often save time generally. Think about these in the same way:
What does it mean when the difference in speed between two objects is 5 m/s?
What does it mean when the average speed of two objects is 6 m/s?

Two buses move down a 100 km road at the same time moving at constant speeds. One bus gets to the end of the road 20 km ahead of the other bus.

What was the distance between the two buses after (a) the faster bus had covered 1/8th of the total distance and (b) the slower bus had covered 1/8th of the total distance?

(a) If you think about this question intuitively then you can solve it pretty quickly.
Since the two buses move at constant speeds and after 100 km the slower bus is lagging behind by 20 km it means that after 1/8th of 100 km the slower bus will be lagging behind by 1/8th of 20 km.
So the answer is 1/8th of 20 = 2.5 km.

On the other hand you can work it out using algebra (another very useful tool in many situations).

Let's call the fast bus's distance dA and the slower bus's distance dB. It is clear from the question that for every 100 km A travels, B travels 80 km and lags behind by 20 km, therefore dB = 0.8dA and the difference in their distance at any time, dA − dB = 0.2dA.

Therefore when dA is 100/8 = 12.5, the distance between is 12.5 × 0.2 = 2.5 km.

(b) In this novel scenario, the algebraic solution is quicker

$$dA - dB = 0.2dA$$

(we need to find dA)

$$12.5 = 0.8dA$$

$$dA = 12.5/0.8 = 15.625$$

so, $dA - dB = 15.625 - 12.5 = 3.125\,km$

Intuitively, if we say the speed of the faster and slower buses in the given time, T are 100 and 80, respectively, to cover 1/8th of the total distance (100/8, i.e. 12.5 km) it will take 12.5/80 = 0.15625T.

In the same time the faster bus would have covered the distance 0.15625 × 100 = 15.625 km. So the difference in distance covered is = 15.625 − 12.5 = 3.125 km.

This question illustrates how having a good grasp of the *concept* of speed more than the formulae can help you resolve these questions.

I have a bucket with a tap at the bottom which empties the bucket at a constant rate of 20 cm³/s. I decide to fill my bucket with water from a tap flowing at a constant rate of 30 cm³/s.

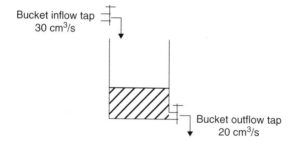

(a) If my bucket takes 5 minutes to fill up, what is the volume of my bucket?
This question is asking you to compare rates. You have the rate of flow into the bucket and the rate of flow out of the bucket. The actual rate at which the bucket is being filled is 30 cm³/s − 20 cm³/s = 10 cm³/s.
Therefore in 5 minutes (or 300 seconds) the total volume that would have communicated is 10 cm³/second × 300 seconds = 3000 cm³.   .

(b) If my bucket has a uniform cross-sectional area of 300 cm² what is the height of my bucket?
This question now calls on your understanding of area and volume, in this case to get the height you need to divide the volume by the area.

Cross-sectional area × height = Volume
Therefore:
Height = Volume/cross-sectional area
Height of bucket = 3000 cm³/300 cm² = 10 cm

(c) I now have this exact same bucket but operating by different rules: the rate of flow from the tap at the bottom of the bucket is not constant but dependent on the height of water in the bucket. It is initially 20 cm³/s but increases linearly by 10 cm³/s for every 1 cm increase in the height of fluid in the bucket. If I start filling the bucket at 30 cm³/s as before (i) what is the maximum height the fluid will reach and (ii) how long will it take to get there?

Now the question has got a bit more complicated; it is asking you to compare two dynamic rates that are dependent on each other. This kind of question does not lend itself very easily to a formulaic approach which you may be used to. This is why it is important to have an intuitive grasp of the problem.

(i)   Initially the net rate is $10 \, \text{cm}^3/\text{s}$, as we have seen. But this changes very quickly as the bucket fills up because the bucket begins to empty at a faster rate.

    Since we know the way the bucket empties we can predict that it would begin to empty at $30 \, \text{cm}^3/\text{s}$ when it reaches a height of 1 cm. At this stage there is a net rate of flow of $0 \, \text{cm}^3/\text{s}$. So it means this is the maximum height the fluid would reach.

(ii) Finding the time it takes to reach the maximum height of 1 cm is a bit trickier because the net rate at which the bucket fills up is not constant. It fills up fast initially but slows down till it gets to zero. What we need is some sort of average rate we can apply. The clue is that the rate of exit from the bucket has a linear relationship to the height of fluid in the bucket.

For simplicity let us take the average rate during that period as $25 \, \text{cm}^3/\text{s}$ (halfway between $20 \, \text{cm}^3/\text{s}$ and $30 \, \text{cm}^3/\text{s}$).

    So all we have to find out is how long will it take to get to the height of 1 cm at a net rate of $(30 \, \text{cm}^3/\text{s} - 25 \, \text{cm}^3/\text{s}) = 5 \, \text{cm}^3/\text{s}$. To know this we need to divide the volume by the rate. The volume at 1 cm height is $300 \, \text{cm}^3$ ($1 \, \text{cm} \times 300 \, \text{cm}^2$).

    So the time taken to fill this volume will be $(300 \, \text{cm}^3/\text{second})/(5 \text{cm}^3/\text{second}) = 60$ seconds.

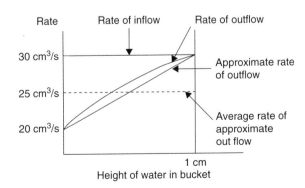

A more complex problem: In addition to the first tap, I open up another tap which fills the bucket simultaneously at 40cm^3/s. Can you draw a graph of (i) rate of fluid exit against time; (ii) height of the bucket against time?

Concentration and other rates

Concentration is a concept you will be familiar with from chemistry but you can also think of it as a kind of rate as the amount of solute changes in a given way with the amount of solution. There a lot of interesting problems that concentrations can throw up.

Billy has two labelled jars, exactly the same in every respect, each containing liquid of equal volume. Jar *A* contains water and Jar *B* contains milk. Billy takes a teaspoon of milk from Jar *B* and puts it into Jar *A*, mixing uniformly. A teaspoon of this new mixture and is then put into Jar *B*. At the end of this process, which of the following is true?

1 The volume of milk in Jar *A* is greater than the volume of water in Jar *B*
2 The volume of water in Jar *B* is greater than the volume of milk in Jar *A*
3 The volume of water in Jar *B* is the same as the volume of milk in Jar *A*
4 The volume of milk in Jar *B* is less than the volume of water in Jar *B*
5 The volume of milk in Jar *B* is greater than the volume of water in Jar *A*
6 The volume of milk in Jar *B* is the same as the volume of water in Jar *A*
7 The volume of milk in Jar *A* is less than the volume of water in Jar *A*

    A *1* and *3*
    B *1* and *4*
    C *2* and *5*
    D *3* and *4*
    E *3* and *6*

This question seems quite simple and straightforward but it does require some thought.

Event 1: milk transferred from Jar A to Jar B.

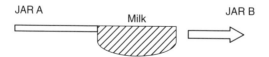

Event 2: milk and water mixture is transferred from Jar B to Jar A.

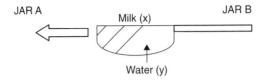

Let 1 teaspoon = 1
Therefore $x + y = 1$
Amount of milk in Jar A $= (1 - x)$
Amount of water in Jar B $= y = (1 - x)$.
Therefore the answer is E.

I take 3 journeys with a taxi company in order to investigate their fare scheme. Below is a table of my three journeys.

Mileage of journey	Total fare for journey
4 miles	£9
12 miles	£24
20 miles	£32

Which of the following fare schemes is most compatible with the provided information?

A £2/mile
B £1.6/mile
C £2 for the first mile and £1 for every mile thereafter
D £3 for the first mile and £2 for every mile thereafter
E £3 for the first mile, £2 per mile for the next 10 miles and £1 for every mile thereafter

This question requires you to interpret a rudimentary table, extract the relevant information and perform a quick search. We have to decide which option is *most compatible* with the information provided.

Option A would explain the second journey 12 miles but will not fit into either of the other two journeys.
Option B would fit into the third journey as £1.60 per mile for a journey of 20 miles will cost £32 but neither of the other options makes sense with this fare scheme.
Option C does not make sense for any of the journeys.
Option D fits the 4-mile journey perfectly but nothing else.
Option E would fit the 1st journey ([1 mile × £3/mile] + [3 miles × £2/mile] = £9) the 2nd journey ([1 mile × £3] + [10 miles × £2] [1 mile × £1] = £24) and the last journey ([1 mile × £3] [10 miles × £2] [9 miles × £1] = £32). Therefore the answer is E.

A quick look at the options will eliminate options *A* and *B* and *C* initially; options *D* and *E* can then be eliminated systematically.

Note that the question asks for the option *most compatible* with the given information. So if the best option was compatible with two of the journeys, that would be the most compatible answer.

> Performing searches is common on the BMAT and UKCAT. Looking at the question broadly and applying common sense will usually help you narrow down your options and save you time.

Integrative processes

A lot of the time on the BMAT, you will be asked to carry out what we could call integrative processes. This is a way of finding the solution that demands you be able to break down or build-up groups or procedures into (from) their component parts.

> There is a peace-brokering conference being held for the leaders of two nations. In attendance are a 20-member delegation from each participant nation and the Conference leader, so 41 people in total. The Conference leader kisses all the delegates once on the cheek while each delegate kisses each member from their own delegation twice and kisses each member from the other delegation only once.

How many kisses were there in all?

This question requires you to select relevant information and build-up (integrate) the total number of kisses from their component parts (noting wherever there might be overlap).

We have to be careful not to trip over ourselves here – we must write down carefully all the parts we want to integrate and approach the problem logically.

First: The conference leader kisses everyone.
Second: There are two sets of kisses between the two groups.
Third: There are two sets of kisses within the groups – 1 set per group.

If we can find the number of each set of kisses, we can find the total number of kisses. It is important to note that there are two sets of kisses between the groups as each group must kiss and also be kissed.

First: The conference leader kisses 40 people once = 40 kisses
Second: Each of the 20 members of group 1 kisses each of the 20 members of group 2 once = $20 \times 20 = 400$

And, each of the 20 members of group 2 now kisses each of the 20 members of group 1 once = 20 × 20 = 400

Third: Group 1: Each member kisses the other 19 members twice = 19 × 20 × 2 = 760

Group 2: Each member kisses others twice = 19 × 20 × 2 = 760. So the total number of kisses = 40 + 400 + 400 + 760 + 760 = 2,360 kisses in all!

How many kisses does each delegation member receive?
Imagine you are delegate:

First you are kissed once by the conference leader = 1. Second you are kissed once by each member of the opposing delegation = 20. Third you are kissed twice by each of the other 19 members of your delegation = 38. Total number of kisses received by a delegate = 1+20+38 = 59.

(This makes sense as 40 delegates each receiving 59 kisses (40×59) = 2,360 kisses in all.)

Properly identifying the component parts makes building the big picture much easier. Make sure to write clearly on paper so as not to confuse yourself.

In a sample population, people either possess gene X, or they do not. 95% of people with a certain Disease A in this sample population possess the X gene. 99% of people with the X gene do not have Disease A. Of the sample population without the X gene, 99.75% do not have the disease.

   If in a sample group 10 people have Disease A, what is the size of the sample population?

A 4000
B 1000
C 1250
D 1100
E 1150

This question is another type of integrative process asking you to breakdown a population into its component parts again noting where there are overlaps. There are two main ways to approach this question: (1) the mathematical approach; (2) the more intuitive approach. We will go through each approach.

1 A more conventional mathematical approach:

Of people with Disease A: 95% have the X gene (X positive)   (1)

                               5% do not have the X gene (X negative)   (2)

Of X positive (+ve) people: 1% have Disease A   (3)

                         99% *do not* have Disease A   (4)

Of X negative (−ve) people: 0.25% have Disease A   (5)

                    99.75% *do not* have Disease A   (6)

People with Disease A = X +ve people (95%) plus X −ve people (5%)

Therefore, of the 10 people with Disease A

               9.5 people are X +ve and 0.5 people are X −ve

The 9.5 people that are X +ve = 1% of total X +ve population (from (3))
Therefore, 100% of X +ve people = 950

The 0.5 people that are X −ve = 0.25% of total X −ve population (from (5))
Therefore, 100% of X −ve people = 200

Total population of sample size = X +ve plus X −ve

                       = 950+200

                       = 1150 (E).

2 A more intuitive approach.
We can see from the question: *In a sample population, people either possess gene X, or they do not.* Let us represent the whole population with a line:

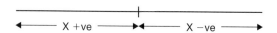

Let the box represent those with Disease A. There is obviously some overlap between those with Disease A and those with and without the X genes.

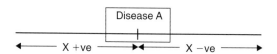

According to the question: *95% of people with a certain Disease A in this sample population possess the X gene.* This is represented in the diagram:

Also according to the question: *99% of people with the X gene do not have Disease A. Of the sample population without the X gene, 99.75% do not have the disease.* This is shown in the diagram below.

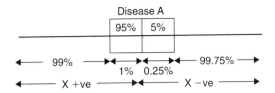

It should be clear from the diagram that 1% of those with the X gene = 95% of those with Disease A. Also, 0.25% of these without the X gene = 5% of those with Disease A. We have thus integrated the information given to form a composite diagram and we have done this intuitively. We can now go on to answer the question.

Number of people with Disease A = 10.

To find the whole population we need to find the people in the population with the X gene and the people in the population without the X gene and add them together.

Since number of people with Disease A = 10.

95% of them = 1% of the population with the X gene = 9.5 people.

Therefore, total number of people in the population with the X gene = 9.5/1 × 100 = 950. Also, 5% of the people with Disease A = 0.25% of people without the X gene. Therefore total number of people in the population without the X gene = 0.5/0.25 × 100 = 200.

Total population = 950 + 200 = 1150 (E).

Analogy
The ability to find similarities between different items or groups of items is in itself a basic skill of problem solving. It may apply to any type of problem; based on words, shapes, graphs or numerical data. The ability to detect analogies requires a combination of different skills and functions we have already looked at in this chapter. You might be asked to determine similarities between entities – anything from numbers, words or graphical data. In these questions, you must first try and work out the entity from a given chunk of information and then try and find it in or relate it to the various options you are given. You might also be asked to determine the similarities between processes. Let us go through a few examples.

The diagram shows a square whose area is a^2

a

a

Which of the following shapes could have the same area as the square?

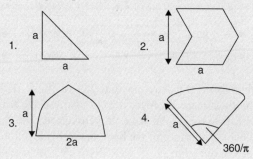

This question tests your ability to spot similarity between shapes using your understanding of areas – the key is to spot how each of the test shapes are similar in size or shape to the square.

Shape 1 (the triangle): It is clearly a half of the square therefore so is its area. You can get the triangle from the square by drawing a diagonal between any two opposite corners of the square. So we know the area of the triangle will be $\frac{1}{2}a^2$.

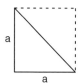

Shape 2: It is possible that this object has the same area as the square, with a chunk of it transferred to another part of the square, so the area is the same. This is shown below.

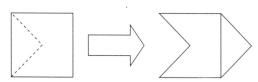

Shape 3: It is more difficult. Here, if you imagine that the base was actually connected to the apex by two *straight* lines, it would form a triangle with area = $\frac{1}{2} \times a \times 2a = a^2$. However, the curved lines make it larger than this, therefore the area will be greater than a^2.

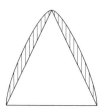

Shape 4: It is a sector. Its area will relate to how large the angle at the apex is, specifically it will be:

(angle/360) $\times \pi r^2$, in this case:

$$\frac{(360/\pi)}{360} \times \pi a^2 = a^2$$

Bus A travelling at 30 km per hour and Bus B travelling at 40 km per hour simultaneously leave from two separate termini 140 km apart. They are travelling towards each other on the same road and therefore meet at some point. Because the difference in distance covered by these two buses in any given time will be 1/3rd of Bus A's distance and since they are travelling toward each other, it must mean the differences between the distances covered must be 1/7th of the total distance covered (i.e. 20 km at the point which they meet).

Which of the following shows an analogous process of reaching the solution?

(a) Buses C4 and C8 travel toward each other from two termini 100 miles apart at 30 mph and 40 mph, respectively. Because the difference in distance covered by these two buses in any given time will be 1/4th of C8's distance and since they are travelling toward each other, it must mean the differences between the distances covered must be 1/8th of the total distance covered, that is 14.3 km.

(b) A car (50 mph) and moped (20 mph) travel towards each other on the same road, starting 140 miles apart. It takes the car 2.8 hours to cover the distance while it takes the moped 7 hours to cover the same distance. The difference in distance when they meet is the difference in distance each of them covers in the mean times, i.e. (7+2.8/2).

(c) Two Bees flying towards each other at the same speed are brought to an abrupt halt when they bump into each other and cover the same distance in getting there because there is no difference in distance covered per unit time.

(d) A car and moped, both travelling at 75 mph, starting 300 miles apart will each cover ½ of the total distance when they meet, i.e. 150 km.

(e) John (walking at 3 mph) and Bill (jogging at 7 mph) move around an 8 mile circuit starting out at the same point but in opposite directions. Per given time, the difference in distance covered by each of them will be 4/7th Bill's own distance, and as they are running in opposite directions on the track, when they meet, Bill would have covered 3.2 km more than John (that is 4/10ths of the total distance).

In any question like this, we first need to establish *what* we are comparing each of the options with – it is the *process* of finding out some measure of the difference in distance covered when two objects meet.

First of all we need to understand the process itself:

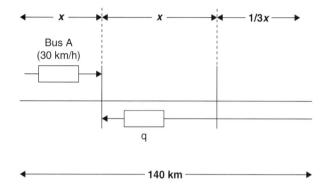

This process uses the fractional relationship of the speeds of the moving object to work out the difference between their distances. It has 3 parts:

1 It first expresses the difference in their distances at any given time as a fraction of the distance of Bus A. For every 30 km Bus A travels, the difference is $40 - 30 = 10$ km; as a fraction of Bus A's distance this is $10/30 = 1/3$ (we could just as validly say that the difference in their distances is ¼ of Bus B's distance).

2 Then, it goes on to relate this difference to the total distance travelled. Lets call Bus A's distance "x". We know that since the gap between them at any time is $(1/3)x$, Bus B must have travelled $x + (1/3)x$.

   Total distance travelled (by both of them) is therefore: $x + x + (1/3)x = (7/3)x$.

   The distance between them, as we have said, is $(1/3)x$. It is clear that this is 1/7th $[(1/3)/(7/3)]$ of the total distance.

3 Finally, it goes on to calculate the *actual* distance this difference equates to when they meet. Since we know that when they meet the total distance covered is 140 km it is now easy to calculate this value since

$$x + x + (1/3)x = 140$$
$$(7/3)x = 140$$
$$(1/3)x = 20 \text{ km}$$

Now look at each of the options.

(a) Here, the difference is expressed in terms of the faster bus (C8), but the calculations based on this are wrong. Therefore, the process is wrong (and therefore not completely analogous).

(b) This option is clearly not using the idea of fractional relationships to reach a solution.

(c) The full process is not needed because it is immediately clear that the difference in distance at any time is 0.

(d) Exactly the same as C, but with the distraction of including a fraction; if you look closely though you will see that the fraction refers to their *individual* distances *not* the difference in their distances (which is 0).

(e) Firstly, do not be thrown by the fact that this is a circuit; since they are travelling toward each other, this is no different from travelling from two ends of the same road (if you like, think of the round-circuit unfurled into a straight line). Here, like in A the difference in their distances is expressed in terms of the faster man, Bill. So, what is the total distance covered by both of them?

(Lets call Johns distance "J" and Bills distance "B".) Just as in the example it is:

$$J + J + (4/7)B.$$

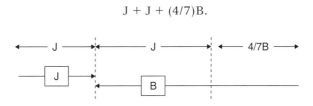

We need to get this in terms of B (as this is the unit of comparison). From the information, J is equal to $(3/7)B$.

Therefore total distance covered $= (3/7)B + (3/7)B + (4/7)B = (10/7)B$

So the difference in distance, which we said was $(4/7)B$ is 4/10ths of the total (this is correctly mentioned in the option).

When they meet:

$$(3/7)B + (3/7)B + (4/7)B = 8$$

$$(10/7)B = 8$$

Therefore

$$(4/7)B = 3.2\,km \text{ (also correctly mentioned in the question).}$$

Therefore, although the expression of difference is first expressed in terms of the faster man rather than the slower man, the overall process after this is almost exactly the same and correct answers are derived, therefore this would be the *most* analogous. (Remember, it is the *process* that you are interested in not the "system" it is based on.)

Applying the analogy . . .

The following table shows sales figures for Henry's food store

Year	Sales
1999	12000
2000	13200
2001	14520
2002	15972
2003	17569.2
2004	19326.12
2005	21258.732

Which of the following competitors showed a similar a pattern of growth in terms of Sales figures?

Charlies'	GoodFood	Organix
500	10000	12000
1700	11000	13000
2900	12100	14500
4100	13310	16000
5300	14641	18000
6500	16105.1	20000
7700	17715.61	23000

Henry's sales shows 10% year-on-year growth, a pattern only seen by GoodFood Sales. Just as in the previous examples, there are two steps to solving this:

First, spot the underlying rule or pattern governing year-to-year change in sales. One way to do this would be initially to see the absolute difference between sales from one year to the next – from this you would see that the difference from year-to-year is not constant, but that it is 10% of the previous year's sales.

Secondly, look for the same or a similar pattern in the options given.

Two tile designs, A and X undergo a standardised modification algorithm, giving rise to two new designs B and Y, respectively.

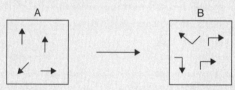

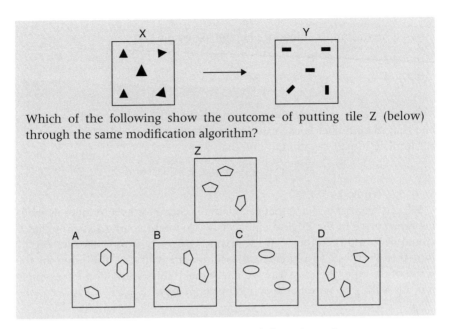

Which of the following show the outcome of putting tile Z (below) through the same modification algorithm?

To determine the pattern, the question to ask here is, "What common process has occurred to both A and X?"

1 Both of the titles have been rotated by 90° in a clockwise direction.
2 In addition, in A the arrows have also gained an extra line, while in X the triangles turn to rectangles.

We can generalise both of these to the fact that the process involves rotation through 90° clockwise and the addition of a line or side.

For Z, only tiles (A) and (B) have undergone rotation in the correct direction and out of these, (B) keeps the same shape whilst (A) forms hexagons (an extra side added), so the answer is *A*.

In some questions involving analogous relationships, determining the analogy is only part of the skill involved. Solving these questions requires the ability to sift through the given information and select that which is relevant. Having done that, you must then find a way to combine the relevant information in order to break the code or discover the rule. You may then be asked to *apply* the process or rule to a novel scenario. In these questions it is particularly important that you fully understand the *scope* and *limitations* of the rule you have found (i.e. do not make unnecessary assumptions).

Have a look at the following example:

The following list shows various codes and their interpretations:

2, 1, 4 = BAD
4, 5, 1, 6 = DEAF
6, 5, 5, 4 = FEED

Based on this information, decode the following:

(i) 6, 5, 4

(ii) 3, 1, 6, 5

From the codes already given it seems that each number stands for a letter and that this number is exclusively used for that letter only. Indeed we can accumulate the information to find that:

$$A = 1, B = 2, D = 4, E = 5, F = 6$$

So 6, 5, 4 would be "FED".

We can see that it seems that each letter is coded for by a number depending on its place in the English alphabet, so we might go on to assume that C would be 3 and therefore that the second code – 3, 1, 6, 5 – reads "CAFÉ" (but this is not an absolutely safe assumption: it lies on the limits of the scope of the rule; the only way we might make this assumption for example is if this is the *only* reasonable option out of many).

The following show the results of some encoded sums, where each letter represents a single digit.

Sum 1	ZO/(Y−Q) = ZO
Sum 2	Y + Q = ZO
Sum 3	Y × Q = OP
Sum 4	Q − (Y − Q) = P

Based on the above information, solve the following encoded sums, giving your answer only in the form of the encoded digits already given:

(i) Y − Z =

(ii) Z × Q =

(iii) Y − Q/P − Q =

To answer this, you first need to decode the information given in the box just like in the previous example (except here we use numbers).

1 ZO/(Y − Q) = ZO: from this (Y − Q) must be 1, therefore Y and Q must be two consecutive numbers from 0 to 9.

2 Y + Q = ZO: since adding Y and Q gives a double-figure digit, they cannot be anything below 7 (if Y and Q were 6 and 5, adding them would give an encoded number of the same digit repeated).

Combining these two facts, Y and Q must be one of:
9 and 8 or 8 and 7 or 7 and 6

3 Y×Q = OP. "O" is a common digit with the previous sum (i.e. adding Y and Q gives a number with a common digit with the multiple of Y and Q). Using our shortlist:

9, 8: $9 \times 8 = \underline{7}2$; $9 + 8 = 1\underline{7}$
8, 7: $8 \times 7 = \underline{5}6$; $8 + 7 = 1\underline{5}$
6, 7: $6 \times 7 = 42$; $6 + 7 = 13$

From this, we can eliminate 6 and 7, thus leaving us with two options:

9, 8: $9 \times 8 = \underline{7}2$ $9 + 8 = 1\underline{7}$
8, 7: $8 \times 7 = \underline{5}6$ $8 + 7 = 1\underline{5}$

4 Q − (Y − Q) = P: since Y − Q = 1, then this tells us that 1 number less than Q is P (which you will notice is also the units digit that is obtained by multiplying Q and Y). The only numbers that fit this are 8 and 7, so Y = 8, Q = 7; (and we can work out the rest from that).

Therefore, the answers to the sums are:

(i) $Y - Z = 8 - 1 = 7 = Q$
(ii) $Z \times Q = 1 \times 7 = 7 = Q$
(iii) $Y - Q/P - Q = (8 - 7)/(6 - 5) = 1 = Z$

Part C: Practice

1 Two jars *A* and *B*, one three times larger than the other but with the same cross-sectional area are filled to the top with water. Water pours out of jar *B* at five times the rate that it pours out of jar *A* until the water levels are the same – at this point 10 ml of water is left in each of the jars. How much water has been obtained from jar *A*?

A 3
B 5
C 7
D 10

2 The combined age of Alex and Lewis is 85. How old is Lewis presently, if Alex was twice the age that Lewis was, when Alex was the age that Lewis is now?

A 30
B 34
C 36
D 38
E 42

3 Billy's grandfather has a rare Zenith Blue stamp in his collection. When issued, this cost twenty-five pence. In perfect condition today, he could sell it to collectors for £5. Assuming the prices of stamps have been inflated by 25% since he purchased it, what percentage profit will he make by selling a perfect stamp to collectors compared to obtaining its current monetary value?

A 125
B 1250
C 1350
D 1500
E 15500

4 What is the largest amount of money you can have in coins and still not be able to give change for one pound?
(The only coins allowed are 1 pence, 5 pence, 10 pence, 20 pence, and 50 pence. One pound is equal to 100 pence.)

5 If there are 20 people at a party and everybody shakes hands with one another once, how many handshakes are made altogether?

A 40
B 80
C 160
D 185
E 190

6 If I sleep-in in the morning, I miss breakfast. If I work until 3 a.m. in the middle of the night, I will sleep-in the following morning. I never sleep-in two mornings in a row. I always sleep-in on Sunday and Wednesday mornings.

It is 3 a.m. in the middle of the night and I am working. Look at the statements and decide which must be true.

   1 It is not Saturday tomorrow
   2 I won't eat breakfast
   3 It is Wednesday or Sunday tomorrow

A 1 only
B 2 only
C 1 and 2 only
D 2 and 3 only
E 1, 2 and 3

7 A car with six doors is shown in the diagram below. It has been custom made, so that upon manually closing one door another door or doors open, if already closed, or close, if already open according to the table below:

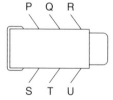

Door Closed Manually	Result
P	Closes both **S** and **U**
Q	Closes **T** and opens **P**
R	Closes **Q** and opens **S**
S	Closes both **R** and **U**
T	Closes **R** and opens **P**
U	Closes both **Q** and **T**

What order of manual door closure will result in all doors being shut?

A (T → P → R → S)
B (S → T → P → Q)
C (P → T → Q → P)
D (S → Q → T → U)

8   At Alabaster College meal tickets for whole-day feeding cost £4.50 each. Each student must purchase a book of 40 tickets. At Marble College students cook for themselves. For use of the kitchen equipment they must pay a fixed charge of £55 per term. Assuming that each term is 6 weeks long and one ticket is used per day, what is the maximum amount, to the nearest 5 pence, that each student at Marble College should spend on average per day in order to be economically better off than students at Alabaster College? (Assume that the students at Alabaster College spend *this* same amount on the extra days not covered by dinner tickets.)

A £3.00
B £3.05
C £3.10
D £3.15
E £3.20

9   Jimmy runs a zoo with zebras, tigers, hyenas and giraffes. He is allowed to keep a maximum of 50 animals. The number of hyenas he is allowed to keep must not exceed twice the number of zebras he keeps. The attendance at the zoo varies in direct proportion to the total number of animals kept and the maximum possible attendance at the zoo is 126.

   What is the number of tigers being kept today, if today he is keeping 4 giraffes and 10 hyenas and the attendance is 76?

A 11
B 12
C 13
D 14
E 15

10   Alice, Bhat, Ching and Daly are friends. Alice lent Ching £30, Bhat lent Ching £10, Daly lent Alice £20 and Bhatt £50. Which of the following actions will clear the debts between them?

A Alice gives Daly £20 and Bhat gives Daly £40
B Alice gives Daly £40 and Bhat gives Daly £30
C Ching gives Alice £10 and Daly £10. Bhat gives Daly £40
D Ching gives Bhat £10 and Daly £40. Bhat gives Daly £40
E Ching gives Daly £30 and Alice £10. Bhat gives Daly £40

11 The antibiotics shown in the table below were rated in a series of trials.

	Trial A	Trial B	Trial C	Total Rating
Ampicillin	X	*	O	350
Amoxicillin	O	O	O	600
Flucloxacillin	*	*	X	200
Methicillin	O	X	O	500

Each trial gave the action of each drug a specific score as indicated by the keys used.

What score did Trial A represent?

A 50
B 145
C 200
D 250
E 550

12 After suffering a stroke, two patients in hospital require intravenous fluids. Based on their weights, it is calculated that they need 2 litres and 3 litres, respectively, given at a steady rate over 6 hours. The volume of 1 drop of fluid is equal to 0.05 ml. If the first drop of both infusions fall simultaneously at exactly midnight:
   (i)   At what time will the two infusions both drop simultaneously again?
   (ii) What is the combined total number of drops that both patients would have received from both infusions when this happens? (Assume that the time it takes for a drop is negligible)

13 Cars A, B and C race from Point 1 to Point 2 and back at constant speeds along an elliptical track. Car A is faster than B and B faster than C. After the start of the race the only time car A and C cross each other, car C has only gone 4/11 of the way from Point 1 to Point 2.
   If car B is moving at three times the speed of car C what fraction of the distance between Point 1 and 2 will car A have covered between passing car B and car C. (Ignore actual bends at both ends of the ellipse which make up a negligible part of the distance from point 1 to point 2.)

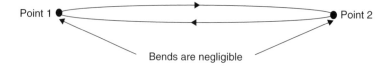

Point 1   Point 2

Bends are negligible

CHAPTER 2

Critical analysis for the BMAT and the UKCAT

Part A: First glance

Many people get a bit confused by the term "critical thinking". It is obvious to most that it involves thinking of some kind but they are not sure what is so critical about it and sometimes assume it is just a fancy way of saying *clever* thinking. The "critical" part of critical thinking refers to arguments. Critical thinking is the thinking that involves and centres around arguments: *understanding and analysing arguments*. It is a Thinking Skill which is an extremely useful thing to be able to do. Critical thinking is very useful in weighing up and comparing conflicting arguments. In science, the arts or politics, wherever you find arguments, you will need critical thinking. Even in everyday life we are constantly evaluating arguments and making choices based on these evaluations.

We are always thinking critically – analysing arguments – we can't help it. But the way we do it is mostly intuitive and implicit, this means it is subconscious and automatic; and that is the problem! We do not explicitly say, "I am going to weigh up the arguments for and against buying that red pair of shoes", or outline the reasons why we don't believe the story about the talking chicken; we just do it, instinctively and implicitly. This is fine when the arguments are rudimentary and fairly obvious. But this instinctive method begins to fall down when we encounter more subtle, even misleading arguments – and you can be sure you will get at least your fair share of these in your exam(s)! To be able to avoid pitfalls and solidly analyse more complex arguments, you must develop an explicit method for analysing arguments, you must begin to articulate many of the processes you already carry out subconsciously and implicitly. This is what we aim to achieve in this chapter.

The skills required for critical thinking are also useful when analysing other kinds of verbal texts other than arguments. They are very helpful in comprehending and analysing passages in general. Candidates sitting either the UKCAT or BMAT are advised to read the *whole* chapter and attempt *all* the questions. Learning the skills required to evaluate arguments will also give you the skills needed to make safe inferences from passages of all sorts.

Part B: The approach

Inference

The first broad skill we are going to consider is deduction or inference. It is the ability to determine what can and what cannot be *derived* from given informa tion. This is the major ability tested on the UKCAT and it forms a part of the skill-set tested on the BMAT, an important point of overlap between the BMAT and UKCAT. In the UKCAT you are provided with stimulus material – a short passage of some kind (not necessarily an argument). You are then asked to determine what can safely be deduced from the passage; in other words what logically follows from the given information. You are also required to determine what definitely does *not* follow and what may or may not follow.

To be able to draw deductions or make inferences, it is useful not only to comprehend, i.e. get a good grasp of the issues discussed but also to pay attention to the details of the passage. Let us consider the passage below, and the statements which follow:

Amplitude modulation [AM] is a technique used in electronic communi-cation. The amplitude of a wave represents the strength of the wave. In AM, changes in the strength of the transmitted signal carries some infor-mation about the message being sent. This could be the loudness of the sound being produced or the brightness of a pixel.

Frequency modulation [FM] on the other hand uses changes in fre-quency of the transmitted signal to carry that kind of information. The strength of the signal is not modified.

AM is more susceptible to noise interference. This is because random electronic signals, which are inevitable, get added to the signal being transmitted along the way and alter its amplitude. As such, it is some-times difficult to determine what the strength of – and therefore the message contained in – a particular signal was when it left the sender, as it has been altered by noise.

For each of the statements (1 to 4) below, decide whether they are true, false or you cannot tell from the information given in the passage.

Statement 1: *Noise is unavoidable.*
The passage says "random electronic signals, which are inevitable" and it also says "as it has been altered by noise". If you combine those two statements in the context of the passage, we can see that random electronic signals is the same thing as noise, so it must follow logically that noise is unavoidable. The answer is *true*.

Statement 2: *FM is better than AM as a technique of electronic communication.*
The passage does not say anything about which is better AM or FM. We might be tempted to think that the FM is better than AM because the passage shows a way in which FM might be better. But this would be an example of a conclusion that is too "heavy" for the reasons given. It may be true, as we have seen, that FM is better but it may also be true that AM is better. We simply don't know, so the answer is *can't tell*. Remember not to let what you actually know interfere with your answer. Your answer should be based only on the information given in the short passage, and nothing more.

Statement 3: *The amplitude and the strength of a wave are equivalent.*
Looking through the passage we can see "The amplitude of a wave represents the strength of the wave." This means that they are equivalent. So the answer is *true*.

Statement 4: *FM is not susceptible to noise interference.*
This is a difficult one. Because we naturally think that since it says "AM is more susceptible to noise interference", it must mean that FM has some susceptibility to noise. But it could also mean that FM has *no* susceptibility to noise. In either case, the quote from the passage would still stand. So the answer is *can't tell*.

Now let's try another example.

> The retail price index (RPI) is considered a measure of the cost-of-living. It takes the price of a basket of specified goods and services purchased by consumers and measures this over time to indicate the level of inflation in a society. The basket may include such services as water rates but does not include investment items such as stocks or shares. Food and energy prices are also always excluded from the RPI. This is due to the fact that the cost of these items are often subject to frequent and large-scale variation which are usually short term; for example the supply of oranges affected by a poor harvest would increase their price for that season. In the UK the RPI is published monthly by the Office for National Statistics.

Statement 1: *One may measure inflation by using the RPI.*
RPI over time indicates the level of inflation. So it is *true*.

Statement 2: *All goods and services are included in the RPI, except energy costs.*
We know food is not included in the RPI, so the statement is *false*.

Statement 3: *If one owns shares in a company, which then rise, one's cost-of-living as measured by the RPI would have also risen as a direct result.*
Well, we know that shares are excluded from the RPI, so they cannot affect it. As such, the statement is *false*.

Statement 4: *The cost of a litre of water is irrelevant to any measure of inflation.*
According to the passage, water rates are relevant to the RPI which itself is
relevant as a measure of inflation. So it is *false*.

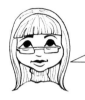

> You must always be *critical* of what you read.
> Always look for a reason why a statement might be
> wrong. That way you won't be caught out by
> difficult statements.

Evaluating arguments

The first set of skills required for critical thinking and on the BMAT is the
ability to understand the mechanics of arguments; what they are, their
components and the relationship between these components. We are going
to find out how to perform these skills – which form the basis of critical
thinking.

What is an argument?

Well, take the two examples below; which one of them is an argument and
which isn't?

> Six million bicycles in Beijing are an enormous burden to the bicycle
> tyre manufacturers when everyone gets a puncture at the same time.

> When the roads are congested in large cities, like Shanghai, it is high
> time to intervene. Congestion charges for vehicles are a good solution
> because they deter vehicles from entering the city. They do this because
> some people will be rather unwilling or unable to pay.

You probably think it is obvious that the second one is the argument. The
question is why?

Well, very simply an argument exists when someone is trying to *make a
point by supporting it*. Firstly, someone must be trying to make a point, that
is to say convince you of one thing or the other and secondly they don't
just do that by stating their point; they go on to try to "prove" it by giving
reasons. This is different from the first example which is simply a statement
which may or may not be true.

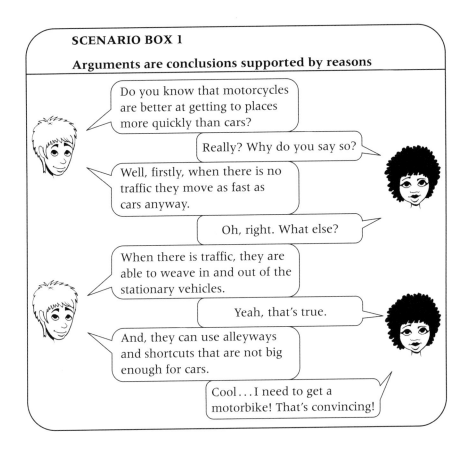

Can you identify which of the following below are arguments and which are not?

> Unlike current abstinence aids, which create violent side effects following alcohol consumption, cognitive therapy alters brain activity associated with reward and pleasure signals.

This statement may look like an argument on initial inspection but it is not an argument. The way we know this is that it is not trying to make a point or convince us of anything. It is simply telling us the difference between the workings of cognitive therapy and current abstinence aids. However, if we changed it to something like this:

> Unlike current abstinence aids, which create violent side effects following alcohol consumption, cognitive therapy is much better because it works by altering brain activity associated with reward and pleasure signals.

It becomes an argument. Previously, it wasn't fighting for anything in particular; instead now it seems to be making the point that cognitive therapy is better than current abstinence aids. What is more, it has given us a reason for this point of view. Remember an argument is not just making a point but giving reason(s) to support it as well.

> Family business is generally not a good type of business to go into. It combines all the tensions of family life with all the stresses of the workplace and is therefore more stressful than regular businesses. The lifetime of family businesses is relatively short, with few lasting beyond the 2nd or 3rd generation. Only 5% of family businesses are still creating shareholder value beyond the 3rd generation.

This is clearly an argument because it follows our rules. It is trying to make the point that family business is generally not a good type of business to go into. It then goes on to elaborate the reasons why. Can you list the reasons given?

> The deregulation of airlines in Europe, which allow any carrier to fly any route, and therefore increase competition resulted in a significant decline in airline fares. This is because with more choice available to the consumer each business has to work harder to gain customers. It is clear that increased competition between businesses inevitably affects consumer-prices.

This again is an argument, a bit more long winded than the last one but it is an argument nonetheless. The point of this argument is the conclusion that increased competition between businesses inevitably affects consumer-prices. To support this point of view the author cites an example from the past.

> The ever-expanding and ever-cheaper market for holidays abroad is certainly a very attractive one, allowing holidaymakers exposure to different environments and cultures. Most holidaymakers find many aspects of long-distance vacations enjoyable, but when things go wrong, this can be stressful.

There's no convincing happening here! You might be tempted to think otherwise because it initially sounds like the groundwork for an argument is being laid. But by the end of it, we can see that the author is not trying to prove a point or convince us of anything in particular, just making an observation.

Breaking down an argument: Parts of an Argument

As we have seen, an argument can be represented in the form:

Argument = Reason(s) $\longrightarrow$ Conclusion

This illustrates the point that in an argument, reasons lead to a conclusion. Reasons are also known as *premises*.

When confronted with an argument the first question you ask should be, "What point is the author getting at?" In other words, what is the conclusion? The way to do this is to ask yourself, "What is the author trying to say? What is the author going to all this trouble to prove?" The next question that should be asked is, "What are the author's reasons? Why does the author hold this view point or why should I be convinced?"

Harry is a medical student. All Medical students have stethoscopes. Harry has a stethoscope.

This is a fairly basic argument. We can rewrite the argument as:

Harry is a medical student *and*
All medical students have stethoscopes *therefore*
Harry has a stethoscope.

So in this case, the argument is quite straightforward – the author is trying to prove to us that Harry has a stethoscope and we can see that two reasons have been used to support this conclusion.

Identifying the Reasons and Conclusions of Arguments

Can you identify the conclusion and reasons in the arguments in the tests below?

Since 1975 many synthetic everyday household chemicals have been banned from being tested on animals. This has been proposed as one reason why cancer rates are increasing because we have not been able to determine their ill effects by animal experiments before common usage. Until these chemicals have been properly tested, only natural products should be used.

Firstly we must ask ourselves what the conclusion is. In this case the conclusion is the last sentence. To confirm we have correctly identified the conclusion we must then go on to pick out the reason or reasons the author is using in attempting to support his/her conclusion.

To make this process easier it is better to re-write the argument in a simpler format. This argument can be re-written like this:

Reason = We cannot determine the ill effects of synthetic chemicals without proper testing on animals, *so* . . .

Conclusion = Only natural or properly tested synthetic products should be used as everyday household chemicals

> A recent news article reported that newly introduced credit card payment methods have cut high street fraud by 13% in one year. However, in the same time period, online banking fraud has increased by over 350% which is totally unacceptable. Since it is easier to police the high street, we should return to the old method of credit card payment to reduce the total fraud overall.

Let us carry out the same process for this argument. Looking for the conclusion, we see again that the conclusion is part of the last sentence. You will find that it is quite common to find the conclusion of an argument near the beginning or the end of the paragraph and this is usually because the conclusion is the climax of what is being said. But we must be careful not to rely too heavily on this fact as it is not always the case.

Having identified the conclusion, we must then go on to see why the author holds this view point. In other words identify the premises (reasons) of the argument. If we re-write the argument, it will go something like this:

Reason 1 = Since the introduction of new credit card payment methods, there has been a drop in high street fraud while online fraud has risen in the mean time, *and since* . . .

Reason 2 = It is easier to police high street banking than online banking, *therefore* . . .

Conclusion = We should return to the old methods of credit card payment to reduce total overall fraud.

In this argument there are two reasons supporting the conclusion. An argument can have as many reasons as possible. Sometimes arguments with many reasons can be difficult to untangle, this is why it is important to be able to analyse arguments by writing them out again simply so one doesn't get lost in the midst of many reasons.

> Obtaining a class II in university examinations is a default state which requires nil or minimal effort while obtaining a class I or class III requires somewhat more effort. This can be seen from the results which show that most people sitting university examinations obtain a class II while only a few people obtain a class I or class III.

Here again is a conclusion backed by a single premise, with a relatively straightforward connection. When we untangle it we might have something like this:

Reason = Most people sitting university examinations obtain a class II, therefore . . .

Conclusion = Obtaining a class II in university examinations requires nil or minimal effort

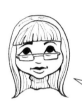

Linkers
Words like "therefore","because", "and so", "as a result", "hence" can be thought of as argument indicators. They are often used to link the premises of an argument to the conclusion. Even if they are not used in the given argument, you can use them to help you effectively break down arguments.

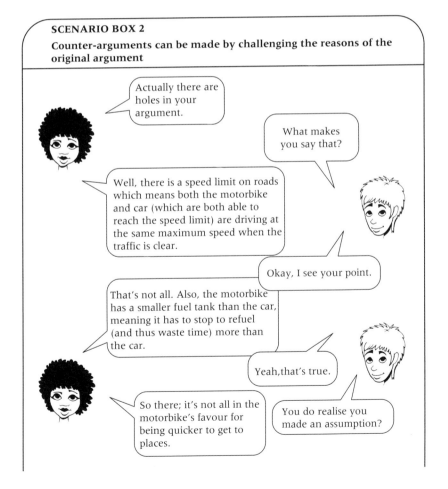

SCENARIO BOX 2

Counter-arguments can be made by challenging the reasons of the original argument

Actually there are holes in your argument.

What makes you say that?

Well, there is a speed limit on roads which means both the motorbike and car (which are both able to reach the speed limit) are driving at the same maximum speed when the traffic is clear.

Okay, I see your point.

That's not all. Also, the motorbike has a smaller fuel tank than the car, meaning it has to stop to refuel (and thus waste time) more than the car.

Yeah, that's true.

So there; it's not all in the motorbike's favour for being quicker to get to places.

You do realise you made an assumption?

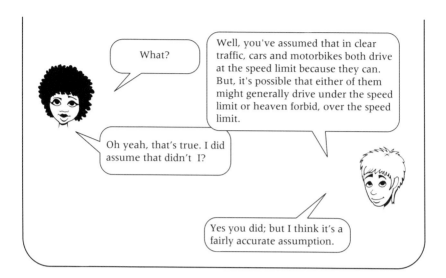

The ways in which reasons relate to conclusions in arguments

> Harry is a medical student. All Medical students have stethoscopes. Harry has a stethoscope.

This is an argument we have come across before. Let's have a further look at it. We know that there are two reasons leading to a conclusion but these reasons do not stand alone. They are not independent of each other. We need both reasons to be able to support the conclusion. We cannot have the argument A or B below:

> A
> All medical students have stethoscopes therefore Harry has a stethoscope.

This argument does not work. The fact that all medical students have stethoscopes *does not* tell us anything about Harry. If we take the argument on its own without any prior knowledge it is a very weak argument indeed.

> B
> Harry is a medical student therefore Harry has a stethoscope.

Although it sounds a bit more plausible that because Harry is a medical student he will have a stethoscope, the argument still does not work.

We can only make sense of arguments A and B if we make certain assumptions. In argument A, if we assume that Harry is a medical student then the argument is fine, while in argument B if we assume that all medical students have stethoscopes the argument makes sense.

In these two cases the author has assumed that we appreciate that either Harry is a medical student (in A) or that all medical students have stethoscopes (in B), so he has failed to mention it. Without these assumptions, what we have is a baseless argument. We will talk more about these kinds of assumptions later in the chapter.

You can have premises working together to support a conclusion.

When you remove one of these reasons, the conclusion cannot be supported by what is left. The argument falls down.

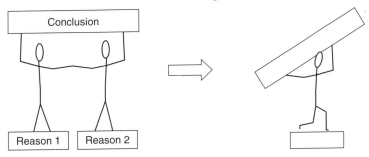

Laura knew her biscuits were poisonous. Laura gave me her biscuit. I heard from Jonathan that Laura wanted to poison me, therefore I think that Laura was attempting to poison me.

This is another argument with premises working together to support a conclusion.

The author concludes that Laura is attempting to poison him/her.

If we break down the argument we have something like this:

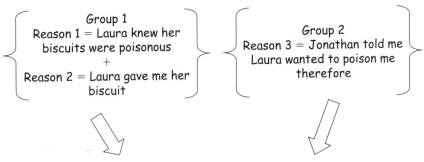

Conclusion = I think that Laura was trying to poison me

You can see here there are two separate groups of reasons which support the conclusion. The author gives three reasons in all for reaching the conclusion that Laura wants to poison him/her. Two of these reasons work hand-in-hand while the third reason works alone, i.e. it is an independent reason.

The way we know that the third reason is independent is that, if left alone it would still be able to support the conclusion.

> I heard from Jonathan that Laura wanted to poison me therefore I think that Laura is attempting to poison me.

Here the third reason alone is able to back the conclusion.

> Laura knew her biscuits were poisonous and Laura gave me her biscuit therefore I think Laura was attempting to poison me.

We have now removed the third reason, and Reasons 1 and 2 are able to back the conclusion. But if we remove either Reason 1 or 2, the argument will fall apart because we have seen that these two reasons work together to support the conclusion. You can see them as *one composite* reason – because effectively they make one reason. If you separate them like *this*:

> Laura knew her biscuits were poisonous therefore I think that Laura was attempting to poison me.

or this:

> Laura gave me her biscuit therefore I think that Laura was attempting to poison me.

Then the argument doesn't really work. This illustrates the concept of *dependent* and *independent* reasons.

An argument can be supported separately by independent premises.

Even if you remove one of the independent premises, the conclusion can be carried by the remaining premise(s).

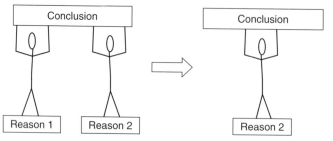

We have seen that reasons can work together or alone in supporting the conclusion of an argument. Sometimes a reason can act as a mini conclusion within an argument. We call this the minor conclusion (or intermediate conclusion).

We have seen that to identify a conclusion we need to look for the main point the author is making or driving at. Sometimes in order to make his main point, an author will need to make a mini point that will back up his main point. This mini point is the mini conclusion.

> To be able to pass the upcoming bill, the constitution requires that the Presidency receives a majority of votes in the 100-man Senate. The news says that the bill has been passed. To be able to get a bill of this sort passed, the President must be loved by the Senate majority leader.

This is an example of an argument with a mini conclusion. We can actually break it down into two different arguments.

Argument 1

Reason 1 = To be able to pass the bill, the presidency needed at least 51 votes from the Senate. And....

Reason 2 = The Presidency got the bill passed, this means....

Conclusion = The Presidency got at least 51 votes from the Senate.

Argument 2

Conclusion (now a premise) = The Presidency got at least 51 votes from the Senate.

Main conclusion = The President must be loved by the Senate majority leader.

We can see that this is actually two arguments tied into one. The author needs the conclusion of the first argument to make his main point. The conclusion of the first argument is called the mini conclusion and the final conclusion is the main conclusion. So it serves as a conclusion in the first argument but as a premise to the main conclusion.

The full argument will look something like this:

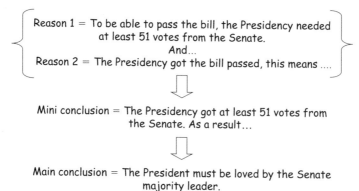

We have seen that in some arguments a mini conclusion acts as a reason for the main conclusion and such arguments might take the form:

Argument = Reasons → (Mini conclusion) → Main conclusion

On your exam, you will usually be asked to identify the major conclusion of the argument but in order to be able to do this effectively it is important to be able to distinguish between the major and mini conclusions.

After identifying the conclusion, you would expect that it would be very easy to identify the premises: since an argument is made up of premises and conclusions, when you remove the conclusion everything left should be your premises. But as you can imagine, this is simply too good to be true and is usually not the case!

Most arguments you will encounter on your exam are part-filled with extra material: this means material that neither serves as premises nor the conclusion. They might help to give you some context or some explanation but sometimes they are not essential to the argument in any way. You must take care not to get tripped up by this and be able to separate the wheat from the chaff.

Figure: The Components of an Argument: A mini conclusion, supported by a premise, and which itself supports the main conclusion, plus some extra parts.

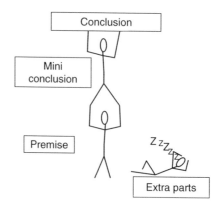

The increased intake of sugar by primary school children is a major cause of the decline in educational achievement seen across the country. Inability of children to sit still and learn means that they underperform at a critical stage in their education setting them up for long-term failure.

This argument shows a combination of different kinds of premises which relate to the final conclusion. Argument components: let's break it down:

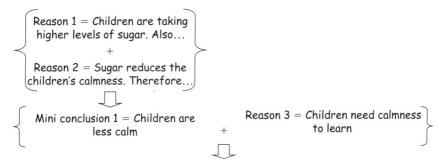

Here Reasons 1, 2 and 3 work together to support the main conclusion – none of them can stand alone (see for yourself if you can make the argument work without one of the three premises). First of all, Reasons 1 and 2 together result in a mini conclusion of their own. This mini conclusion is omitted in the argument because it is *assumed that we can figure this out*. Then Reason 3 together with (the mini conclusion of) Reasons 1 and 2 provide support for another mini conclusion which then results in the main conclusion.

So, in this argument we actually have two mini conclusions, although only one of them is explicitly stated in the argument. You can have several mini conclusions in an argument, each one dependent on the previous one like this:

Argument = Premise → Mini Conclusion → Mini Conclusion → Mini Conclusion → Main Conclusion

There is a problem with arguments structured in this way. If you have a conclusion supported only by a chain of mini conclusions then your argument is not as strong as it looks. This is because if one of the links in your chain of reasoning is successfully broken then your whole argument falls down.

For example, if I can prove that sugar does not reduce the calmness of children (i.e. their ability to sit down and learn) then I can destroy the whole argument just by breaking one of the links. If sugar does not reduce the calmness of children then it does not reduce their ability to learn and so does *not* set them up for long-term failure. We will see later that one of the ways we can weaken an argument is to disprove one of its premises. This argument looks quite strong initially because it has several reasons but a deeper look has revealed that it isn't that strong since it is a string of dependent reasons. If the argument had some other reasons that stood alone, i.e. supported the conclusion independent of the other reason, then the argument might still be standing.

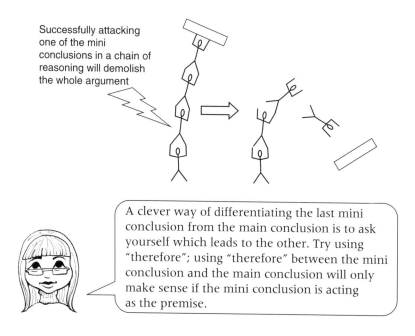

Successfully attacking one of the mini conclusions in a chain of reasoning will demolish the whole argument

A clever way of differentiating the last mini conclusion from the main conclusion is to ask yourself which leads to the other. Try using "therefore"; using "therefore" between the mini conclusion and the main conclusion will only make sense if the mini conclusion is acting as the premise.

Assumptions

Sometimes not all the premises in an argument are explicitly stated. The author might fail to explicitly state one of his premises because it is assumed.

Harry is a medical student therefore Harry has a stethoscope.

This is an argument we have seen before. It is incomplete. If we had no other information and took it at face value, then it does *not* make sense. I *do not* know what medical students have or do not have, neither do I know what Harry has or does not have, I only know that Harry is a medical student so how can I conclude that Harry has a stethoscope? It really is a silly argument. But this is only because we are being very strict and rigid.

On the other hand, if I were to assume that the author is sane, knows what he is talking about and is generally good at making coherent arguments, i.e. if I were to give the author the benefit of the doubt, then the argument *could* make sense. It would make sense if I assumed that all medical students have stethoscopes. Then the argument would go:

All medical students have stethoscopes, Harry is a medical student there-fore Harry has a stethoscope.

I have added a reason to make the argument complete. If we give the author the benefit of the doubt then we say that he or she took it for granted that "All medical students have stethoscopes" and so failed to mention it in the argument. Such a reason that is taken for granted (i.e. assumed) and therefore not explicitly stated in the argument (i.e. implicit) is called an *implicit assumption* for obvious reasons.

An implicit assumption is key to the integrity of the argument.

If the assumption is successfully disproved, the argument does not stand.

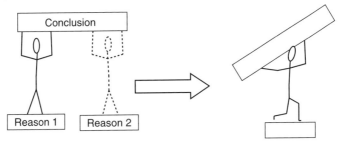

Violence is only acceptable if one is faced with a direct threat because then it is done in self-defence.

What is/are the underlying assumptions?
To be able to pick out the implicit assumption in an argument, you have to break the argument down to its bare bones:

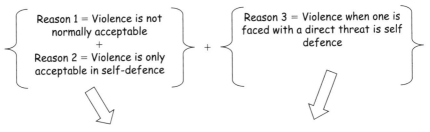

It should be clear that Reason 1 is the implicit assumption. The argument has something missing without Reason 1. We have seen that an implicit assumption or underlying assumption is a premise that is not stated in the argument but necessary for the argument to fully make sense. Reasons 2 and 3 are stated in the argument but Reason 1 is taken for granted and is not stated. Without Reason 1 the argument is incomplete.

Beware: An implicit assumption cannot be stated in the argument because if it is, it is no longer implicit!

> The increased intake of sugar by primary school children is a major cause of the decline in educational achievement seen across the country. Inability of children to sit still and learn means that they underperform at a critical stage in their education setting them up for long-term failure.

This is an argument we have seen before. Breaking it down:

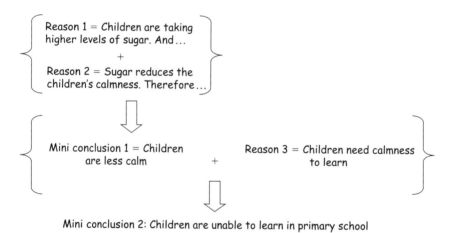

Here, the argument is slightly more complicated. The assumption may not be immediately obvious. We have broken it down and yet it seems to make sense without any possible assumptions being added.

This is because we generally tend to read assumptions into arguments. We take it for granted, just like the author has, that the reason is not actually stated in the argument. If we look a bit more closely at the argument and the breakdown we have done, you might notice a missing link:

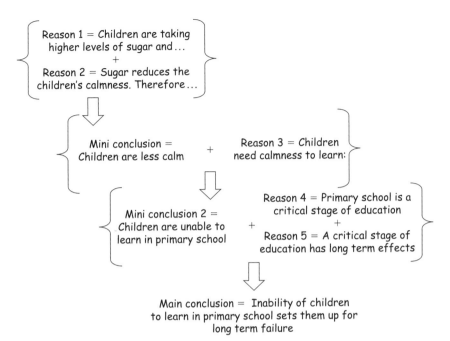

Reasons 4 and 5 are essential to the argument – without them the argument does not stand up to real scrutiny. In fact you could think of more assumptions in this particular argument.

When an assumption is essential to the argument, like this one, it *underlies* the point being made, i.e. it is an *underlying assumption*.

SCENARIO BOX 3

Attacking underlying assumptions

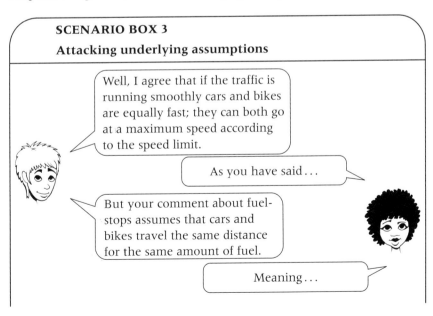

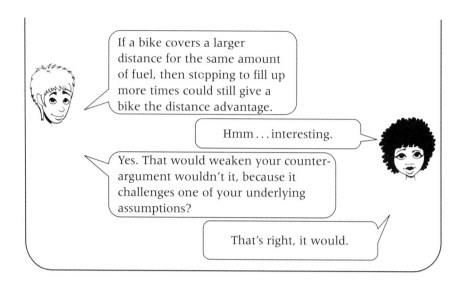

If a bike covers a larger distance for the same amount of fuel, then stopping to fill up more times could still give a bike the distance advantage.

Hmm... interesting.

Yes. That would weaken your counter-argument wouldn't it, because it challenges one of your underlying assumptions?

That's right, it would.

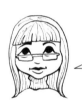

In order to find the implicit assumption in an argument, ask yourself, "Does the author fail to state it?" If the answer is, "yes", then ask yourself, "Is it essential to the argument?" If the answer again is "yes" then you are probably looking at the implicit assumption.

Precipitation levels have been very high recently in Zagarabia. As a result wheat farmers have seen a downturn in produce, their only means of sustenance, which explains the increase in the rate of poverty among the wheat farming community.

Reason 1 = Rainfall levels have been very high recently. Also...
+
Reason 2 = Wheat produce levels are down due to high rainfall. Plus...
+
Reason 3 = Farmers depend on wheat as a means of earning a living

Conclusion = Wheat farmers are earning less of a living i.e.
poorer due to the high rainfall levels

Can you spot the assumption from the breakdown? If you look at the argument more closely, you will find that it can be broken down in a better way.

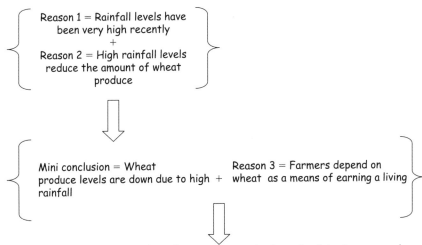

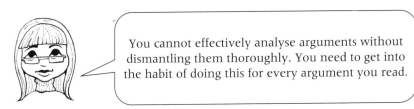

We have now done a more thorough job of breaking down the argument and it becomes a bit clearer that there is a missing reason – Reason 2 – which is the implicit assumption.

It is *vitally important* to become efficient at dismantling arguments because that is the key to answering Critical Thinking questions on the BMAT. The better you are at it, the more obvious the answers will seem to you.

> You cannot effectively analyse arguments without dismantling them thoroughly. You need to get into the habit of doing this for every argument you read.

Drawing your own conclusion

So far we have tried to extract the conclusion of the argument from the stimulus material provided. The arguments contained the conclusions and we were just meant to pick apart the argument and then identify the conclusion.

Not all arguments you will come across on your exam will have the conclusion written in the text. You will be given some incomplete arguments that do not contain conclusions. In situations like this you will be asked to provide the conclusion that follows logically from the premises provided, i.e. to *draw your own conclusion* from the stimulus material. This is a type of inference. You can infer what conclusion should follow from a set of reasons.

It is not only the conclusions of arguments that can be inferred from an argument. As we have seen, anything that follows logically from a piece of given information can be inferred. This might be the conclusion of the argument as we have seen, or even an implicit assumption.

It is important to note that you will be asked to provide a safe conclusion, or what can most safely be inferred. What it means for your conclusion or inference to be safe is that your conclusion can be based *totally* on the information provided. In other words, your conclusion can be trusted to derive directly from the information. The common mistake here is to use additional information to make an inference. This is wrong as you are asked to determine what can safely be inferred from the *information given*.

For example, scientists have to draw conclusions from the results of their experiments. These must be derived solely from the results of their experiments and what is known to be true. If it doesn't, for example if they overgeneralise or jump to conclusions without sound evidence the conclusions reached are deemed unsafe because they may be wrong. This is the meaning of a safe conclusion.

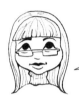

Deduction
A process of reasoning in which a conclusion follows necessarily from the premises presented, so that the conclusion cannot be false if the premises are true.

Strengthening and weakening arguments

The other important set of skills you need is to be able to show the weaknesses or strengths of arguments or to try and strengthen them or weaken them yourself. In order to do these you need to be able to understand how to break down arguments, which we have done already.

Flaws in arguments

The flaws in an argument are basically of two types. Either because the reasons themselves are false or inaccurate or the logic is faulty, i.e. even though the premises may be true, they do not logically lead to the conclusion. By the same token, to weaken an argument, you can either disprove one or all of its main premises or introduce new evidence to show why it may be wrong, or show that it has faulty logic.

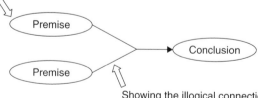

The privatisation of the police force in Belgravia is absolutely ridiculous. It shows that this government is totally incompetent. You cannot privatise the police force because the police force is an arm of government and should be under the control of the government. Giving private individuals control of the police force means that they wield as much power as the state and this reverts us to anarchy.

This argument actually seems quite forceful on initial reading but we need to break it down to be able to look for flaws.

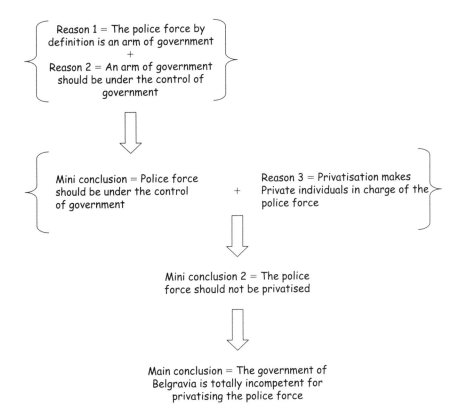

We have broken down the argument into its different parts and what you can see here is that it starts off quite well but doesn't end so well. The glaring flaw here is that of faulty logic. We all might agree that the police force should not have been privatised but how does that lead us to conclude that the government is *totally incompetent*? The author has gotten carried away here. This is a classic mistake – where the conclusion is too big for the premises.

The conclusion can be too heavy   The conclusion may be properly
for the reason(s) used to support it   supported by adding reason(s)

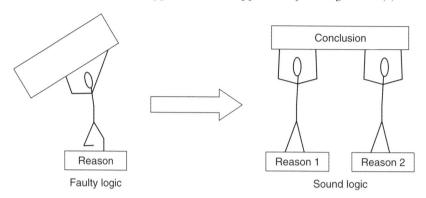

How would this argument change if the conclusion said "The Belgravian government may be incompetent?" This would mean that the conclusion would be "lighter" and so could be carried by the premises. It then becomes plausible that the Belgravian government may be incompetent (if we assume that what it is doing is one sign of incompetence). The wording drastically changes the argument.

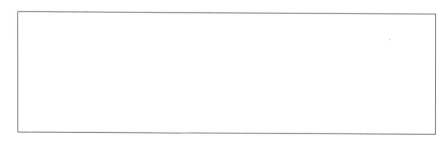

First of all, can you make a reasonable attempt at breaking down the argument?

This is another example of an argument showing weak logic. It may be true that blondes generally are very good at mathematics (if we assume that is the author's point) but I simply cannot reach that conclusion purely on the basis of students in my school. Even if the top maths students in my school are blonde, it doesn't mean that blondes everywhere are good at maths. The blondes in my school may be atypical or the non-blondes in my school may be particularly bad at maths, making the blondes seem better than they are. There might be no relationship whatsoever between the colour of your hair and your ability at mathematics.

All medical students have stethoscopes. Harry has a stethoscope. Harry is a medical student.

First of all, can you make a reasonable attempt at breaking down the argument?

This argument is superficially similar to one we have come across previously. It is another example of faulty logic. The fact that all medical students have stethoscopes does not mean that everyone with a stethoscope is a medical student. So, even though Harry has a stethoscope, it does not mean he is a medical student.

Common Errors of Logic

Unsafe Conclusions: We have had a brief look at unsafe conclusions. A conclusion is unsafe when it cannot be trusted to be true even if the premises are true. It doesn't mean it isn't actually true. For all we know it may eventually turn out to be true, but we cannot accept it at the moment based on the evidence provided. A safe conclusion is *always* true *if* the reasons are *true*.

Cause versus Correlation: Sometimes when two factors increase or decrease together, there is the temptation to think that one is causing the other. Let us take an actual example. In the past there was evidence to show that the more alcohol you drank the more likely you were to get lung cancer. This was because scientists found a correlation between alcohol consumption and lung cancer. A correlation simply means that when one factor goes up or down, the other factor goes in the same direction. So people who drank loads of alcohol tended to get lung cancer, while people who drank little or nothing at all, were much less likely to get lung cancer. Now, what did that mean? Some people began to say that alcohol was causing lung cancer. This was an unsafe conclusion.

When there is a correlation between two factors, one of three things could be happening

1   *Coincidence*: In this case, there is no link between the two factors. We all understand the concept of coincidence – a chance happening. Someone wearing the same top as you at a party doesn't mean he/she knew what you were going to wear – it was a coincidence. So the link between alcohol and lung cancer could have been a simply coincidence, nothing more to it. So even if there was a correlation (i.e. the reason was true) the conclusion could still be wrong, hence unsafe.

2   *Indirect link*: On the other hand, there could be an indirect link between two correlated factors. Not that one factor causes the other but that they are both linked to a third factor which may be affecting them both. In the case of alcohol and lung cancer, the third factor was smoking. People who smoke tend to drink alcohol. The more they smoked the more they tended to drink. So, we now know that it was actually the smoking causing the lung cancer, an invisible link between the two factors.

3   *A direct link or causation*: Finally it may be that one factor is actually causing the other. But how do we know which is causing which? Why did people assume that the alcohol was causing the lung cancer and not the lung cancer somehow causing people to drink? Without any further evidence, it isn't possible to determine which is the cause and which is the effect. Can you think of some factors that can help determine the direction of the causal relationship?

Extrapolating a trend: Another common error of logic is to assume that because something has been happening a certain way, it will continue to happen that way for no other reason than that it has been happening that way.

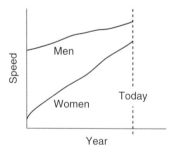

Above is a graph that illustrates the way the average speeds of male and female athletes has changed over the last few decades. What can we safely say about these speeds in the future? Are women athletes going to become faster than men athletes?

Over-generalisation: This was the problem with the example about the blondes and mathematics. It is a common error. Because something applies to a member of a group, doesn't mean it applies to everyone in the group. If upon picking up his first orange, a foreigner concludes that all oranges are yellow – it is an unsafe conclusion. It does not follow that because one member of a group has a certain characteristic, all members do. The argument about the Belgravian government is another example showing how easy it is to jump to conclusions.

Researchers have recently discovered that over the last 50 years colour TV ownership has increased. Over the same time period there was a 2000% increase in people speaking French as a second language. Colour TV ownership should be encouraged as this adds to the nation's French language skills.

Break down the argument:

This is a classic example of confusing correlation with cause. It concludes that the increase in French language skills is due to colour televisions because we have seen increases in both of them over the same time period. As we have seen, this conclusion is unsafe – it cannot be trusted. It may simply be a coincidence, in which case there is no link between the two things. It might be that, it is actually because people are learning French that they are buying colour TVs, maybe to watch French programmes. It may be that buying colour TVs makes people learn French like the argument actually concludes. The point is we just don't know. Because we cannot be sure about this conclusion based on the premise given – the conclusion is deemed unsafe.

Weakening arguments
Sometimes you are asked to weaken an argument. This is broadly similar to finding the flaws in an argument. In this case, you actually have to suggest

something that can be done to make it weaker. The main ways you can weaken an argument are:

1 If you could disprove one or more of the reasons given for the argument – preferably a *cardinal* reason.
2 If you can show that the logic is faulty.
3 If you can provide additional reasons of your own that oppose the argument.

We have already seen examples of faulty logic. Let us take a look at how one might attack the premises themselves.

> Alcohol-related crime and alcohol-induced illnesses can be decreased by increasing the legal minimum age for buying and consuming alcohol from 18 to 21 years. If people are banned from drinking until the age of 21 they are much more likely to adopt more mature drinking habits. Also if people start drinking later they would have fewer years to accumulate the medical risks. It would also allow the popular culture to change to a more sophisticated approach present in continental Europe.

Let's break down the argument:

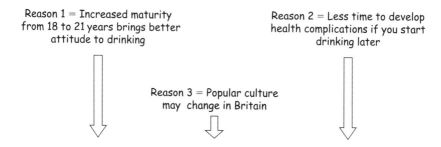

Reason 1 = Increased maturity from 18 to 21 years brings better attitude to drinking

Reason 2 = Less time to develop health complications if you start drinking later

Reason 3 = Popular culture may change in Britain

Conclusion = Poor health and crime linked to alcohol can be reduced if we raise the legal drinking age from 18 to 21 years

If I were to *successfully* show that actually, people's attitude to alcohol and drinking does not change between the ages of 18 and 21, then I have disproved Reason 1 and thus weakened the argument. Remember that the argument has other independent reasons holding it up but is now weaker than before. Even when an argument is logically intact, you can weaken it by attacking one of its reasons.

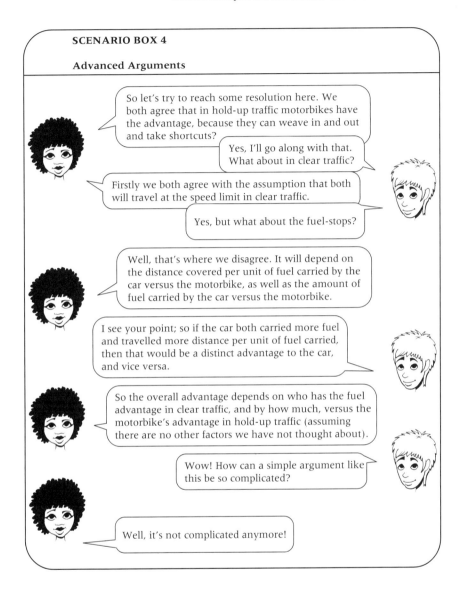

SCENARIO BOX 4

Advanced Arguments

So let's try to reach some resolution here. We both agree that in hold-up traffic motorbikes have the advantage, because they can weave in and out and take shortcuts?

Yes, I'll go along with that. What about in clear traffic?

Firstly we both agree with the assumption that both will travel at the speed limit in clear traffic.

Yes, but what about the fuel-stops?

Well, that's where we disagree. It will depend on the distance covered per unit of fuel carried by the car versus the motorbike, as well as the amount of fuel carried by the car versus the motorbike.

I see your point; so if the car both carried more fuel and travelled more distance per unit of fuel carried, then that would be a distinct advantage to the car, and vice versa.

So the overall advantage depends on who has the fuel advantage in clear traffic, and by how much, versus the motorbike's advantage in hold-up traffic (assuming there are no other factors we have not thought about).

Wow! How can a simple argument like this be so complicated?

Well, it's not complicated anymore!

Part C: Practice

In this section you are provided with questions to practice. It is important to:

(a) Do all the questions (whichever exam you are going to sit).
(b) Make sure you dismantle each argument before answering the question asked and *write down* your argument – breakdown clearly and fully.
(c) Make sure you arrive at *your own* answer before looking at the options.
(d) *Write down* your reason(s) for rejecting each answer option you decide against.

(e) In addition to answering the question(s) asked make sure you also determine: (1) the conclusion of the argument, (2) any implicit assumptions,
(3) any assumptions that are *not* essential to the argument, (4) any flaws
in the argument and (5) ways to weaken/strengthen the argument.
(f) Finally, after attempting all these questions, go back over the chapter and
try to break down all the arguments used more thoroughly (if possible).

1 Family business is generally not a good type of business to go into.
It combines all the tensions of family life with all the stresses of the
workplace and is therefore more stressful than regular businesses.
The lifetime of family businesses is relatively short, with few lasting
beyond the 2nd or 3rd generation. Only 5% of family businesses are
still creating shareholder value beyond the 3rd generation.

Can you breakdown the argument into its parts, showing how they relate to
each other?

2 Increased competition between businesses inevitably affects consumer-
prices. Deregulation of airlines in Europe (allowing any carrier to fly
any route) for example resulted in a significant decline in airline fares.

Which one of the following if true most seriously weakens the above
argument?

A Some routes saw an increase in carriers while others saw a reduction in
participating carriers.
B Deregulation of airlines in Europe saw a reduction in the average number
of carriers flying most routes.
C The surplus of carriers wishing to fly some routes led to partnership-deals
between carriers, where, in many cases fare-prices were fixed.
D The decrease in average airline fare-price was not universal, with many
routes showing increases of up to 100%.
E Deregulation in Asia which increased competition did not affect airline
fares at all.

3 Global warming is a major concern to most scientists, yet political action has not responded in the same way. Many industrialised nations fear that capping carbon emissions will harm their powerful economies and increase unemployment. Developing countries believe it is against their interests to stop burning cheap and readily available fossil fuels to build up their economies, in the same way the industrialised countries did before them.

Which of the following could be used against developed countries?

A The existence of tough emission limits will increase innovation and provide alternative fuels.
B Global warming is more important than terrorism.
C Action must be taken now to see measurable effects in a timely manner.
D Unemployment levels have increased and decreased in the past without capping emissions.
E Fossil fuels are in diminishing supply.

4 The theory behind the use of ID cards seems reasonable enough. The idea that it will help fight crime such as tax evasion, welfare fraud and terrorist activity as well as increasing police powers is indeed compelling in an age where information is as potent a weapon as any conventional police tactic. Proponents of ID cards have added that their use could be voluntary rather than compulsory and add further that they would help all carriers by enabling more efficient receipt of government services. However, it is merely an impractical and fundamentally flawed tool, not to mention its high cost of implementation. ID cards would simply add further burden to law-abiding citizens whilst technology-savvy criminals escape through the inevitable loopholes. In order for ID cards to be effective in their primary purpose, they would have to be universal. The only way to make them universal is to make them compulsory. The inevitable fines and other types of punishment that will result (for those who do not comply) will only worsen matters.

Which of the following best expresses the conclusion of the above argument?

A Although results of ID cards are useful in principle, their use in practice is unlikely to achieve the desired aim.
B The idea of ID cards is not as simple as it seems.
C The implementation of ID cards is fraught with difficulties.
D Proponents of ID cards are wrong.

5 The basic argument for control of guns, that general access to guns causes higher crime, is contradicted by the facts and by reason. Lower murder rates in many foreign countries don't prove that gun control works. Many of these foreign "role-models" do not actually have gun control laws. Thousands of children are said to die annually in gun accidents but this is misleading, as gun accidents involving children have actually been quite low in recent times. Moreover it is more practical in protecting society, to allow access to guns and monitor who obtains them rather than a blind ban on gun possession.

Which of the following best expresses the main conclusion of the above argument?

A Gun possession is an inalienable right of citizens.
B Ownership of guns is not related to increased crime.
C As gun crime rises, opposition to gun ownership rises.
D Lower murder rates are not related to gun control laws.
E General access to guns should be allowed.

6 Purchasing a lottery ticket in the knowledge of the miniscule chance of winning is almost justifiable. But how many people actually do truly *understand* how small their chance of winning is? In many ways, buying a lottery ticket in the hope of being the jackpot winner is like throwing money away, and these games are no more than an extra burden on the poor, who are in most need of the money but who can least afford to play.

Which *two* of the following are implicit assumptions of the above argument?

A Many people buying lottery tickets are poor.
B Most people don't understand how small a chance they have of winning.
C Many poor people do not play the lottery.
D Most of the money from purchasing the lottery ticket goes to the Government for discretional use.
E Most of the money from buying the lottery ticket does not go to charitable causes.

7 With the increasing emergence of viable alternative-energy technologies, the 21st century may be marked by a move away from fossil fuels equal to their large-scale adoption during the industrial revolution. The environmental damage wrought by the use of fossil fuels is extensive, and many people argue, unsustainable. This combined with the

increasing pressure brought to bear by an issue that is now high on the political agenda means that the vast majority of people and their governments will adopt alternatives if available. Alternatives such as the use of sunlight, wind and other renewable forms of energy have, slowly but surely, become transformed from experimental models to commercial realities. This heralds the dawn of a new energy revolution in renewable energy.

Which of the following best expresses the main conclusion of the above argument?

A Fossil fuels will become less popular in the near future.
B This century may see a drastic undoing of the industrial revolution.
C Alternatives to fossil fuels are becoming more popular and this will fuel the energy revolution.
D This century may see a large-scale move away from fossil fuels as a source of energy.
E Renewable forms of energy such as sunlight and wind are the future of energy.

8 The link between smoking and lung cancer is well known. What is not fully understood, however, is how the pattern of smoking influences the risk of lung cancer. Take, for example two patients who present to their GP with symptoms warranting investigation for possible lung cancer. The first, Mr J smoked everyday for the last 22 years. The second, Mr L has smoked only on alternate days for the last 44 years. One would expect the risk of having lung cancer to be the same for both men, but it is Mr L who has now developed cancer. This is thought to be because the action of the toxins in cigarette smoke persists even after initial exposure. This case conclusively shows that the number of years smoked has as much of a bearing on the risk as the amount smoked.

Even if the evidence is correct, which of the following shows that the conclusion is unsafe?

A It may be the case that Mr L and Mr J did not smoke the same number of cigarettes on average per day as each other.
B It may be the case that certain genes which make people to start smoking later also increase cancer risk.
C It may be the case that Mr L lived in a city with more second hand smoke (which can cause lung cancer) than Mr J.
D It may be the case that in the next five years Mr J will have developed cancer.

E It may be the case that Mr J and Mr L share the same susceptibility for developing cancer.

F It may be the case that Mr L is older than Mr J and this is why he has developed cancer.

---

9 A recent news article reported that newly introduced credit card payment methods have cut high street fraud by 13% in one year. However, in the same time period, online banking fraud has increased by over 350% which is totally unacceptable. Since it is easier to police the high street, we should return to the old method of credit card payment to reduce the total fraud overall.

Which of the following are underlying assumptions of the above argument?

A High street fraud is made easier by the new payment methods.
B Online banking is too difficult to police.
C The high street fraudsters have moved to online banking fraud.
D Technological progress has to be halted in order to reduce crime.
E The increase in online fraud brought about by the new payment method outweighed the decrease in high street fraud over the same period in absolute terms.
F The increase in online banking fraud was because of the new payment method.

---

10 Which *two* of these statements are equivalent?

A All sheep with GSS have amyloid plaques
B All sheep free of GSS do not have amyloid plaques
C All sheep with amyloid plaques have GSS
D All sheep with amyloid plaques do not have GSS
E None

---

11 The ever-expanding and ever-cheaper market for holidays abroad is certainly a very attractive one, allowing holidaymakers exposure to different environments and cultures. Yet at the same time, the whole process of ever more elaborate "holidaymaking" can be a self-defeating task. Even before the destination is reached, long queues, unruly passengers, and "sardine" seating on aeroplanes can be, if anything, highly stressful. On reaching the destination, further complications such as language difficulties and an unaccustomed diet may exacerbate rather than alleviate any physical and psychological strain one may have.

Which of the following best describes how the short statement relates to the argument?

Most holidaymakers find many aspects of long-distance vacations enjoyable, but when things go wrong, this can be a stressful.

A Lends support
B Paraphrases one of the arguments main premises
C Neither challenges nor supports the argument
D Challenges one of the arguments main premises
E Summarises the main conclusion

> **12** When the health of the world is at stake, such as during the SARS epidemic and with the threat of a bird flu pandemic, it may be permissible for the international community to punish uncooperative governments to ensure its collective survival.

Which of the following is an implicit assumption of the above argument?

A Punishment of governments by the international community is not normally acceptable.
B Threats such as the SARS epidemic and bird flu could affect any country.
C The health of a nation's citizens is the most important aspect of government.
D Uncooperative governments may be punished by the international community for other reasons.
E Punishment may not involve military action.

> **13** The population of some countries is actually in negative growth. This means that year on year there are fewer babies born. The standard of living has also increased year on year which means that the elderly are living longer. These two facts mean that there is an inversion of the previous demographic picture: where formerly there were more workers than dependents the opposite is now the case. The workforce of the future will be strained and unable to support the number of dependents. One solution is to raise the retirement age. Another is to increase immigration.

Break down the above argument – showing all the reasons (including implicit ones) and how they relate to each other and any flaws. How might you attempt to strengthen/weaken the argument?

14 Genes do not play as important a role in who develops breast can-
    cer as most people think. The presence of mutations in some genes,
    such as BRCA, are known to lead almost inevitably to the develop-
    ment of the disease. However, the number of cases positive for this
    gene mutation are rare. Furthermore, even well established factors
    such as family history, prolonged exposure to oestrogens and previ-
    ous benign breast problems account for less than half of all cases. On
    the other hand it has been increasingly shown that external envi-
    ronmental factors such as food and medication play a more impor-
    tant role. A high-carbohydrate diet for example, seems to increase
    the risk by raising insulin levels, and excessive stimulation by insulin
    is known to be a trigger for cells to grow abnormally. Other dietary
    factors such as alcohol, fruit and vegetables as well exposure to cer-
    tain chemicals can affect risk.

Break down the above argument – showing all the reasons (including
implicit ones) and how they relate to each other and any flaws. How might
you attempt to strengthen/weaken the argument?

15 The presence and activity of theme parks is a good indicator of the
    economic success of a developed nation. In South Korea, economic
    crisis led to a 25% fall in attendance at "Lotte World", its largest
    theme park. On the other hand (in developing nations) supermarket
    attendance rates are much more reliable an indicator as this tends
    to be relatively stable, with attendance at individual supermarkets
    strongly influenced by their specific marketing strategies. This can
    be explained by the simple phenomenon of rational spending: the
    less income people have, the more they cut back on additional
    spending such as leisure pursuits, whereas spending on day to day
    commodities is preserved.

Break down the above argument – showing all the reasons (including implicit ones) and how they relate to each other and any flaws. How might you attempt to strengthen/weaken the argument?

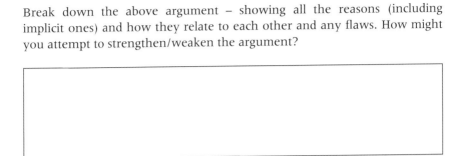

For questions 16 to 21 below, read the passages and answer the questions which follow. For each question state if according to the passage the question is True, False or Can't tell.

16 Seahorses are a species of fish all belonging to the genus *Hippocampus*. The biologically curious feature of the seahorse is that it is the male of the species which becomes "pregnant" – carrying the eggs which the female deposits into a nurture pouch on the front of the male seahorse's body. Here they remain for around three weeks, visited daily by the female until the time for birth.

One might expect with such a departure from convention that other gender roles would be also reversed for example the female to initiate and be pre-eminent in courtship rituals; this is not so. The male takes on this role in the normal manner seen in other species.

Sexual monogamy seems to exist between seahorse pairs at least in the same breeding season. All males and females seem to be programmed to reproduce at the same time, thus limiting the availability of partners to the unpaired.

1 Many seahorse species exist, all belonging to the genus Hippocampus.
2 Females are not required after laying the eggs, since the males carry and nurture the eggs until birth.
3 Once mated, seahorses are monogamous for life.
4 During the breeding season, it is difficult for unmated seahorses to find mates.

17 Paintings by the first human beings were done in caves. Cave artists produced pigment for the colours from rocks and minerals. Black pigment could be made from ground charcoal. White pigment was made from kaolin or chalk. Kaolin comes from the weathering of feldspar, a constituent of granite and other igneous rocks. Granite also consists of quartz and mica. These constituents give granite its

whitish colour. Red pigments were derived from haematite (iron oxide, also known as red ochre). Novel pigments could be produced by the action of heat by some tribes.

Although the majority of minerals used were easily discovered, some had to be mined. We know that ochre mines, for example, existed in Africa and were in action over 40,000 years ago.

1 Cave artists knew that pigments could be obtained from rocks and minerals.
2 Igneous rocks are a source of white pigments.
3 Red ochre pigments come from haematite.
4 Not all pigments which were used were found as raw materials.

18 Around 800 A.D. the first castles in western Europe were built. Approximately 300 years later castle building in northwest Europe reached its peak. Early "castles" were built of timber. These usually consisted of no more than a building situated on the top of a mound of earth. These so-called "motte-and-bailey" castles were usually developed by their later owners: the timber building being replaced by stone – the "keep".

The strategic position atop the hillock was maintained, but the new "castle" usually had the addition of surrounding stone walls as well as stand-alone buildings for living and keeping livestock. As sieges were usually anticipated, a miniature society would usually exist inside the castle walls, with a well, for water supplies, animals for food and a chapel for prayers.

1 The first castles were built around 1200 years ago.
2 Castle building in northwest Europe started to decline after around 1100.
3 Stone "keeps" were not part of original timber motte-and-bailey castles.
4 People could survive in a castle even if it was under siege, for several weeks, even years.

19 The tarantella is a traditional Italian dance originally of the lower working classes but popularised in aristocratic London circles in the 18th century. The German novelist Johann Goethe described it involving three peasant girls who would alternate between the dance and making music with castanets and a tambourine when tired. This form is unlikely to have been the same as that which contemporary London couples would recognise.

The origin of the dance is not known although there are some stories and the name does suggest a clue. In popular legend the dance is associated with tarantula spiders (hence the name). One possible explanation is that the bite of certain tarantula spiders would cause the victim to convulse and "dance around" uncontrollably. Another related story is that having been bitten, the victim would dance in this way in order to avoid harmful effects of the poison.

1 The German novelist Goethe used to dance the tarantella.
2 Once bitten by the tarantula spider, victims dance around uncontrollably.
3 Several stories give us the origin of the name of the dance.
4 Other dances such as the flamenco, tango and charlston are all similar to the tarantella.

20 There is much encouragement for us to eat at least five portions of fruit and vegetables per day. But what exactly is a fruit? Botanically there is a precise definition: a fruit is a ripened ovary of a flowering plant, and includes the seeds which are embryonic plants. Hence a fruit is a vessel for the dissemination of a plant's seeds. This precise definition includes foods which one may ordinarily think of as a vegetable, for example the tomato.

This leads us to consider how we classify fruits and vegetables outside the formal language of botany, and one discovers that it has a lot to do with how these foods are used in cookery. Fruits are usually served as a desert (e.g. apple pie) since they are considered to taste sweet. So although technically a tomato meets the botanical definition of a fruit, we call it a vegetable because it does not fit with our everyday usage of the term fruit.

The word vegetable however has no scientific meaning and indeed any part of a plant which is eaten can be considered a vegetable. Even non-plants, such as mushrooms (which are scientifically classified as fungi), are included.

1 The botanical classification of fruits is ambiguous.
2 All vegetables are savoury.
3 Cookery and Botany do not agree on all aspects of classifying edible produce.
4 A fruit may also be a vegetable.

21 Reality television is a type of television programming characterised by unscripted scenes or situations, usually dramatic or at least funny. It also depicts actual events and uses "ordinary" people instead of

professional actors. It is not a new phenomenon, documentaries and the news, for example, fall under this category. What most people refer to when they speak of reality TV is the recent (since about 2000) explosion in the number of "reality shows" which throws a mix of people together purely for "entertainment" purposes and with no other particular goal in mind.

Reality shows in many ways serve as today's replacement for the secrets-based shows of the past such as Magic shows; where the audience was always left wondering as to the reality of what their senses perceived.

1 Reality shows are a type of television programming.
2 Reality television is a new phenomenon.
3 Reality shows have recently seen an increase in popularity.
4 Reality shows have no point to them.

Some useful definitions

Cogency: The quality or state of being convincing or persuasive: *The cogency of the argument was irrefutable.*

Critical thinking: The mental process of actively and skillfully conceptualising, applying, analysing, synthesising, and evaluating information to reach an answer or conclusion.

Explicit: Fully and clearly expressed or demonstrated; leaving nothing merely implied.

Implicit: Implied or understood though not directly expressed.

Logic: The study of the principles of reasoning, especially of the structure of propositions as distinguished from their content and of method and validity in deductive reasoning.

Premise: A proposition supporting or helping to support a conclusion. A reason.

Validity: Containing premises from which the conclusion may logically be derived: a valid argument. Correctly inferred or deduced from a premise: a valid conclusion.

CHAPTER 3
Scientific knowledge and application for the BMAT

Part A: First glance

Section 2 of the BMAT is "knowledge-based", testing the core knowledge requirements for the advanced study of biomedical sciences. The subjects examined are:

- Biology
- Physics
- Chemistry
- Mathematics

The knowledge requirements for this section are defined by the National Curriculum: up to GCSE level (Key Stage 4) Double Science and Higher Mathematics.

This is by no means meant to be a comprehensive review: we have been selective, focusing on high yield topics – areas that commonly cause difficulty (as reflected in the subject balance). It should be read carefully – as the points are made succinctly and are easily missed if in a hurry.

Instead, we have focused on exactly the angles from which you should expect BMAT questions: less emphasis on knowledge per se but more on the *implications* and therefore the *applications* of this knowledge. This should help you in answering the questions, "why?" and, "so what?" The questions at the end of the chapter are integral to its use – aiding thought about general implications and acting as a springboard for further study.

We hope to push you to think in directions and to depths you might not have considered previously and which your regular exams do not, thereby aiding your preparation for the BMAT.

Finally, in addition to knowledge and understanding, the requisite skills for applying these principles in novel situations overlap with those required for Section 1.

Part B: High yield topics: Subject summaries

Biology

Biology: Humans and other animals

Nutrition and digestive system: General principles

The purpose of the digestive system: to break down complex macromolecules into simple molecules which are absorbed. These simple molecules are "building blocks" which allow the synthesis of more complex molecules required for growth and respiration. The most important mechanism for doing this is by digestive enzymes.

Main food group		Basic unit
Carbohydrate	→	Glucose
Protein	→	Amino acids
Fat	→	Fatty acids and glycerol

Enzymes in digestion
Enzymes: General properties

- *Specificity*: only work for specific reactions.
- *Catalytic*: speed up the rate of reaction without themselves being changed.
- *Variable activity*: enzyme activity (therefore reaction rate) changes under different conditions (pH, Temperature).

Structure, especially of the active site, is crucial to function; if the structure is changed, the enzyme will not work. This may happen by: (i) genetic mutation in the gene coding for the enzyme (ii) denaturation (at high temperature or outside the pH range).

   This means that the activity level of an enzyme varies with changes in the conditions (pH, temperature, the absence of "inhibitors" of the enzyme and the presence of enough substrate); the highest activity level occurs when all the conditions are optimum.

Denaturation = irreversible change to structure.
Inactivation = temporary change depending on change in conditions (normal activity resumes when the conditions are changed back).

Key enzymes and sites of action

Site	Secretions	Key enzyme	Effect
Mouth	Saliva	Amylase	Starch → Maltose
Stomach	Gastric acid	Pepsin	Protein → Amino acids

Site	Secretions	Key enzyme	Effect
Duodenum	Pancreatic juice	Amylase	Starch → Maltose
		Trypsin	Protein → Amino acids
		Lipase (and others)	Fats → Fatty acids (FAs) and Glycerol
	Bile		Large fat droplets emulsified into smaller droplets.
Ileum		Enzymes at surface of villi (e.g. maltase, sucrase, lactase)	Remaining undigested molecules (especially the disaccharides) digested to glucose, amino acids, FAs and glycerol before absorption, e.g. Maltose → Glucose.

Digestive system

Key functions

Mouth: Mechanical digestion of large food particles.

Oesophagus: Transport of food bolus to stomach.

Stomach: Further mixing; production of *gastric acid* for pepsin (protein digestion).

Duodenum: *Pancreatic juice* and *bile* marks the beginning of the main enzyme-based *digestion* to take place.

Ileum: *Absorption* of digested products (*villi* maximise the surface area for doing this).

Large bowel: Absorption of *water* (formation of solid faeces).

Rectum: Storage of faeces before egestion.

The different parts of the GI tract can be thought of as compartments, each with slightly different functions and each providing an optimum environment for that function.

Think about the composition of food at different points in the digestive system. At the mouth there will be largely undigested food with some partially digested carbohydrates; at the stomach there will be in addition some further protein digestion; in the small intestine more and more food will become digested and in addition absorption of this digested food begins.

Circulatory system: Generally

We need a circulatory system because diffusion is inefficient over distances greater than 1 mm. Single celled organisms obtain all the substances they require by the process of diffusion.

We must use a flow system that requires energy to get things where we need them faster.

Circulatory system: Blood

The main purpose of the blood is for rapid *transport*: of heat, cells, nutrients and hormones and other molecules to all parts of the body. *Cells*: *Red blood cells* (carry Haemoglobin) for oxygen transport; *White cells* (for defence against pathogens); *Platelets* help blood to clot, therefore prevent blood leaking at sites of damage to blood vessels.

Oxygen transport and the O_2-dissociation curve:

Oxygen transport by Haemoglobin (Hb) depends on the concentration of oxygen available at the alveolus. The available oxygen at the alveolus is generally on the shallow part of the graph, so that small falls in the available oxygen at the alveolus (pO_2) will hardly cause a change in the oxygen content of blood. Whereas, in the tissues, the pO_2 is at the steep part of the curve so allowing oxygen to move from the haemoglobin to the tissues readily. This means as blood enters deoxygenated parts of the body it will off-load the oxygen quickly.

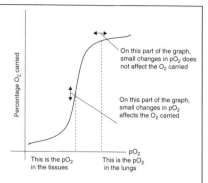

On this part of the graph, small changes in pO_2 does not affect the O_2 carried

On this part of the graph, small changes in pO_2 affects the O_2 carried

This is the pO_2 in the tissues

This is the pO_2 in the lungs

Percentage O_2 carried

pO_2

Vessels: Artery – arteriole – capillary – venule – vein

	Function	Structure	Blood flow	Lumen
Arteries	*Perfuse* (carry blood to) tissues	Thick-walled, *elastic* to withstand *high pressures*	*Pulsatile*	Narrow
Veins	Drain blood *away* from tissues	Thin-walled with *valves*	*Low pressure,* slow	Wide

Circulatory system: Heart
The heart is, effectively, two pumps – the Right side for oxygenating blood (sending blood to lungs) and the Left side for perfusing the rest of the body (therefore larger, thicker-walled left ventricle).

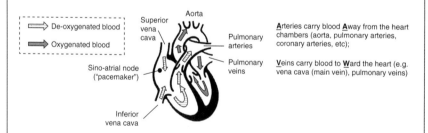

De-oxygenated blood

Oxygenated blood

Sino-atrial node ("pacemaker")

Superior vena cava

Inferior vena cava

Aorta

Pulmonary arteries

Pulmonary veins

Arteries carry blood **A**way from the heart chambers (aorta, pulmonary arteries, coronary arteries, etc);

Veins carry blood to **W**ard the heart (e.g. vena cava (main vein), pulmonary veins)

The heart beat is controlled by a "pacemaker" – the sinoatrial node (at the Right atrium); this generates electrical activity which spreads, first through the atria (causing atrial contraction), then through the ventricles (causing ventricular contraction). The atria and ventricles work one after the other – when the atria are contracting, the ventricles are relaxed, and vice versa – this allows the smooth flow of blood around the heart.

Communication systems: Generally

A single-celled organism performs all its functions using one cell.

As humans we have division of labour, with different systems performing different functions.

In order to work as a whole we need communication between systems to integrate their functions.

The two main communication systems in humans are chemical (hormones) and electrical (nervous system).

Nervous system: Generally

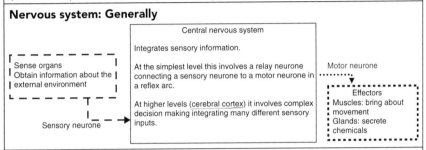

Central nervous system

Integrates sensory information.

At the simplest level this involves a relay neurone connecting a sensory neurone to a motor neurone in a reflex arc.

At higher levels (cerebral cortex) it involves complex decision making integrating many different sensory inputs.

Sense organs Obtain information about the external environment

Sensory neurone

Motor neurone

Effectors
Muscles: bring about movement
Glands: secrete chemicals

Eyes

The eye is a sense organ. The receptors are rods and cones in the retina. The optic nerve is a collection of all the sensory neurons from the retina.

The purpose of the eye is to precisely focus light rays onto a tiny area on the retina (the fovea).

This involves refraction (bending) of parallel light rays to make them converge onto a single point at the fovea. Most refraction is done by the cornea; the lens is used for fine-adjustment. A short, fat lens will refract more powerfully than a long thin lens.

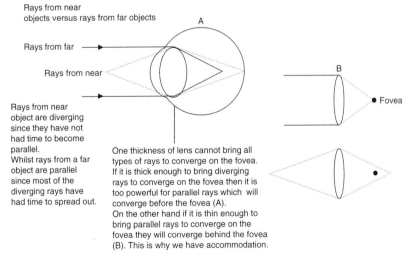

Rays from near objects versus rays from far objects

Rays from far

Rays from near

A

B

• Fovea

Rays from near object are diverging since they have not had time to become parallel. Whilst rays from a far object are parallel since most of the diverging rays have had time to spread out.

One thickness of lens cannot bring all types of rays to converge on the fovea. If it is thick enough to bring diverging rays to converge on the fovea then it is too powerful for parallel rays which will converge before the fovea (A). On the other hand if it is thin enough to bring parallel rays to converge on the fovea they will converge behind the fovea (B). This is why we have accommodation.

The amount of light rays entering the eye is controlled by the pupil – in the dark the pupil will dilate (expand); in bright light it will constrict (become smaller).

Hormones: Generally

Hormones are blood-borne chemical messengers released by endocrine glands directly into the blood stream which travel to parts of the body, and bind to specific receptors on cells to bring about various effects.

Advantage: widespread changes on many cells and organs simultaneously.

Disadvantage: widespread activation of a system means effects can go out of control.

Negative feedback: ensures the system is tightly-controlled (negative feedback means high levels of a hormone act as a "brake" to prevent further production). This is a key mechanism ensuring "homeostasis" (the maintenance of stable environment within the body).

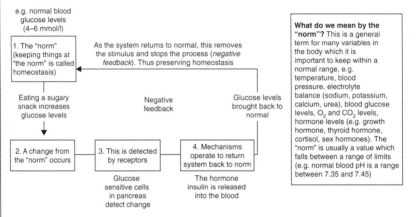

What do we mean by the "norm"? This is a general term for many variables in the body which it is important to keep within a normal range, e.g. temperature, blood pressure, electrolyte balance (sodium, potassium, calcium, urea), blood glucose levels, O_2 and CO_2 levels, hormone levels (e.g. growth hormone, thyroid hormone, cortisol, sex hormones). The "norm" is usually a value which falls between a range of limits (e.g. normal blood pH is a range between 7.35 and 7.45)

Make sure you know the hormones produced by the main endocrine organs (pituitary, thyroid, adrenal, pancreas, ovary and testis) and their effects.

Insulin

Insulin is an important example of a hormone.

Main functions: maintain homeostasis of blood sugar; promote growth.

Produced by: pancreas (which is able to sense high sugar levels).

Action: promotes uptake of sugar from blood by liver and muscle cells. Muscle cells use it to grow, liver cells store it as glycogen.

Diabetes: A condition of high blood sugar when there is one of two problems:
1. Not enough insulin is produced.
2. Cells cannot respond to insulin and therefore cannot take up glucose.

Hormones and fertility

The main sex hormones are

Oestrogen and Progesterone (in females): these promote the development of the female sex organs, regulate the menstrual cycle (production of eggs), bring about changes in the mother in preparation for birth.

Produced by: Ovaries (progesterone also produced by placenta).

Testosterone (in males): promote the development of the male sex organs and the production of sperm.
   Produced by: Testes.

Menstrual cycle	*1st half:* Oestrogen for ovulation (release of the egg).

Menstrual cycle
Normally lasts 28 days, day 1 = first day of menstruation
It can be divided into 2 parts:
1st half (leading up to ovulation) "oestrogenic" (high oestrogen, low progesterone)
(*Ovulation*: half way through, approximately day 14)
2nd half (after ovulation) "progestagenic" (high progesterone, low oestrogen)
Think of the first half as the "build-up" of hormones (oestrogen) which *builds* the womb lining and leads to the release of the egg ("ovulation"). After ovulation, the womb-lining must be *maintained* for pregnancy, in case the egg is fertilised (progesterone).

1st half: Oestrogen for ovulation (release of the egg).
2nd half: Progesterone prepares the womb lining.

- If the egg is not fertilised, the remnant "corpus luteum" deteriorates and stops producing progesterone (so the womb lining breaks down).
- If fertilised, the corpus luteum continues to be stimulated to produce progesterone (to keep the womb lining intact).

In pregnancy, high levels of both oestrogen *and* progesterone are produced.

Breathing
Breathing (or "ventilation") comprises movements generated to inflate (draw air into) and deflate (push air out of) the lungs. Think of the thoracic (chest) cavity as a closed space with the lungs inside (like a balloon in a jar). The diaphragm and intercostal muscles change the volume of this space and create a pressure gradient which cause the lungs themselves to change volume. As the lungs expand or deflate, this creates a second pressure gradient, causing air to move in or out.

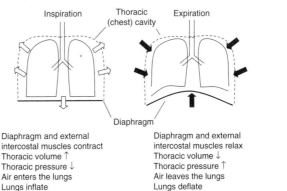

Inspiration   Thoracic (chest) cavity   Expiration

Diaphragm

Diaphragm and external intercostal muscles contract
Thoracic volume ↑
Thoracic pressure ↓
Air enters the lungs
Lungs inflate

Diaphragm and external intercostal muscles relax
Thoracic volume ↓
Thoracic pressure ↑
Air leaves the lungs
Lungs deflate

Aerobic and anaerobic respiration

There is a difference between respiration and breathing. Breathing is the physical exercise of taking air into the lungs (ventilation), respiration is a cellular process.

Aerobic respiration is a series of oxidation reactions of sugars, resulting in the production of energy (in the form of ATP). The main by-product of this is CO_2.

When the oxygen supply is limiting, anaerobic respiration can be used – this results in the production of lactic acid.

Excretion: the kidney

The kidney's function is to remove unwanted chemicals from the blood. The way it does this is to allow most of the molecules in the blood to enter the kidney's tubules (which lead to the bladder) and then pick out only the good, useful molecules thus allowing all the unwanted, bad and strange molecules to leave the body via urine.

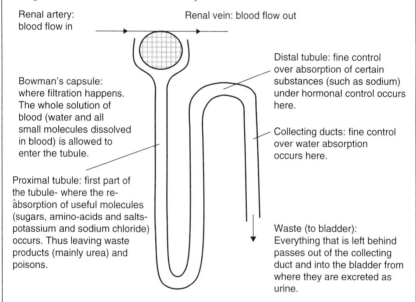

Renal artery: blood flow in

Renal vein: blood flow out

Bowman's capsule: where filtration happens. The whole solution of blood (water and all small molecules dissolved in blood) is allowed to enter the tubule.

Proximal tubule: first part of the tubule- where the re-absorption of useful molecules (sugars, amino-acids and salts- potassium and sodium chloride) occurs. Thus leaving waste products (mainly urea) and poisons.

Distal tubule: fine control over absorption of certain substances (such as sodium) under hormonal control occurs here.

Collecting ducts: fine control over water absorption occurs here.

Waste (to bladder): Everything that is left behind passes out of the collecting duct and into the bladder from where they are excreted as urine.

The volume and composition of urine produced (compared with that of the blood) can therefore tell us about how well the kidney is functioning. A *low volume* of urine suggests that filtration is not adequate – either because of a fault with the glomerulus or because the blood supply to the kidney is impaired.

A *dilute* urine with high salt suggests that salts and water are not being reabsorbed (i.e. a fault with the tubules and collecting duct).

Skeleton and muscles

Movement occurs at joints.

The direction of possible movements depends on the type of joint.

In order to move a joint in a particular direction, one muscle contracts, while its antagonist relaxes.

The speed and force of the movement depends on the force of contraction (and strength) of the muscle acting on the joint.

Ligaments and tendons are known as *connective tissue*.

Ligaments connect bone to bone while tendons connect muscle to bone.

Often, spinal reflexes activate one muscle and inhibit its antagonist simultaneously to bring about a quick reflex movement.

Antagonistic muscles move the joint in opposite directions.

Biology: Variation, inheritance and evolution

Inheritance generally

Genes are the code that determine the structure and function of living things. In humans they are carried on 46 chromosomes, which come in 23 pairs. Each pair of chromosomes carries the same types of genes (except the X and Y chromosomes) – a pair of genes of the same type are called "alleles". Inherited alleles may be dominant or recessive:

- A dominant allele will always express its effect (phenotype).
- A recessive allele will only express its effect if there is no dominant allele (gene of the same type) on the other chromosome.

Sex determination Combination of X/Y chromosomes determines sex. Sperm cells can either have X or Y chromosomes. Egg cells can only have X chromosomes. Therefore sperm cells (i.e. the father) determine the sex of the child.	XY = male. XX = female.

Variation generally

Variation refers to *differences* in characteristics between individuals. These may be *genetic* or *environmental*.

Genetic causes of variation and mutation

Differences in the type of genes people have cause differences (variation) in their *phenotype*.

Variation is a characteristic of *sexual reproduction* which involves:

(a) different combination of genes contributed by the mother and father
(b) differences in sex cells produced by each parent (due to meiosis).

Biology: Life processes

Chromosomes/DNA

Chromosomes are clusters of DNA.

DNA (deoxyribo-nucleic acid) molecules are molecules which, in different sequences "code" for the production of various proteins and enzymes, which control the function of the cell.

The part of DNA coding for a specific protein is called a *gene*.

Cell division: Mitosis and meiosis Mitosis: Regular cell division that allows a cell to replicate itself. *All* chromosomes are copied, so that the new cell gets an exact copy of the DNA. Meiosis: Only involved in production of *sex cells* (*sperm and ova*). Pairs of chromosomes divide from each other, producing *non-identical* cells.	The genetic make-up of each sex cell produced by the same person is different, as meiosis produces sex cells with different combinations of chromosomes. This allows for variation in offspring produced.

Chemistry

Chemistry: Atoms and molecules

Nucleus, protons, electrons

Sub-atomic particles; protons are positively charged, electrons are negative, neutrons are neutral. The protons and neutrons (nucleons) are inside the nucleus and make up the bulk of the atom. Electrons with a negligible mass circle the nucleus. The mass number of an element denotes the relative atomic mass.

For an element, E

$E_{Z=\text{atomic (proton)}}^{A=\text{mass number}}$
number

Bonding

All atoms (except noble gases) are found in combination with other atoms. This is because the most stable configuration, from an energy standpoint, is when atoms have full outer shells. Bonding enables stability.

Covalent bonds

Electrons are shared in pairs between atoms. Found between atoms of non-metallic elements and in compounds (usually between non-metals). Every shared pair of electrons = a covalent bond.

Covalent compounds, e.g. O_2, CO_2: usually non-conductors, low melting point (m.p.)/boiling point (b.p.) when present in molecules, high m.p./b.p. when giant structures.

Ionic bonds

Electrons are transferred between atoms to form ions. The positive and negative charges of ions attract one another strongly. Ionic bonding is usually between reactive metals and reactive non-metals, e.g. Na^+Cl^-, $Cu^{2+}SO_4^{2-}$.

Other types of bonding

Metallic bonding: Every metal atom donates electrons to a common "sea of electrons" in which the cations are held.

Polymers consist of very long molecules in which atoms in the chain are joined by strong covalent bonds.

Chemistry: Changing materials

Solubility

Solubility of a solute in a solvent is expressed in grams of solute per 100 g solvent.

Chemistry: Chemical reactions

Acids, alkalis, bases

pH scale $(0 \rightarrow 14)$ shows how acid or alkaline a solution is. pH 7 = neutral.

pH is a measure of the concentration of H^+ ions

High $[H^+]$, high acidity, low pH, $\rightarrow 7 \rightarrow$ low $[H^+]$, low acidity, high pH.

- Acids must be dissolved in water to show their characteristic properties, i.e. $H^+(aq)$

Base = a chemical that reacts with an acid to produce a salt and water only. 　Alkali = a soluble base. 　Alkalis produce OH^-(aq) when they dissolve in water. 　Neutralisation: when an acid + alkali reacts to form water.	• All alkalis are bases; not all bases are alkalis. • Metal oxides and metal hydroxides are bases.
Oxidation, reduction During oxidation and reduction there is always movement of electrons. *Oxidation*: The combination with oxygen or loss of hydrogen (or electrons). *Reduction*: The loss of oxygen or gain of hydrogen (or electrons). A reducing agent allows reduction to occur to another substance by removing oxygen or giving hydrogen. A reducing agent is therefore oxidised itself. An oxidising agent allows oxidation to occur to another substance by donating oxygen or removing hydrogen.	• Remember "*OIL RIG*". • **O**xidation **is l**oss (of hydrogen/electrons). • **R**eduction **is g**ain. • *Common oxidizing agents*: oxygen, chlorine, hydrogen peroxide. • *Common reducing agents*: hydrogen, carbon, sulphur dioxide
Equations and formulae Atoms of different elements have different masses. One mole of any substance contains the same number of particles (the Avogadro number). 　The relative atomic mass (RAM) is a way of comparing masses of elements relative to one another. Amount (mol) = mass (g)/RAM Amount of solute (mol) = {Volume of solution (cm^3)/1000} × concentration of solution (mol/dm^3)	Avogadro's number $= 6 \times 10^{23}$ $1 l = 1000\,cm^3 = 1\,dm^3$ $mol/l = mol/dm^3 = mol\,dm^{-3}$.
Conservation of mass Mass and energy are conserved in reactions. Any net difference is exchanged as heat with the surroundings.	
Reversible reactions Dynamic equilibrium applies Le Chatelier's principle. If conditions change, the equilibrium shifts to *counteract* the change. Catalysts do not alter the position of equilibrium – just speed up the rate of reaching equilibrium.	Changing conditions may include: temperature, pressure, removal of product.
Reactivity series A list of metals in order of reactivity. This is drawn up after observing whether or not a metal reacts with air, water and acids and how vigorously. *Highest Reactivity* K, Na, Li, Ca, Mg, Al, C, Zn, Fe, Sn, Pb, H, Cu, Ag, Au, Pt 　　　　　　　　　　　　　　　　　　　　　*Lowest Reactivity* More reactive metals can displace less reactive metals from its compounds. $2Al + Fe_2O_3 \rightarrow 2Fe + Al_2O_3$ *or* $Cu + AgNO_3 \rightarrow Ag + Cu(NO_3)_2$	

Reaction rates Factors affecting rate include: concentration of a reactant in solution (or pressure of gases) (the more particles which can collide in a given space); temperature (the faster particles collide, and with more energy); surface area of reactants (increased reacting surface of particles); presence of a catalyst (lowering activation energy). Collision theory can explain rate of reactions: in order for a reaction to occur: (1) particles must meet, (2) they must meet with enough energy to overcome the activation energy.	Concentrated acid reacting with a powdered substance at high temperature with addition of a catalyst = fast rate (all increase the likelihood of particles meeting, with enough energy to react).
Catalysts Allow reactions to occur at lower temperatures (and thus reduce costs). Are not used up (so can be recycled – but can be poisoned by impurities (and inactivated)). May not be available for every reaction – different reactions require different catalysts.	Enzymes are biological catalysts – may not work in extreme conditions (the protein structure can irreversibly denature).
Exothermic/endothermic Energy is transferred when chemical reactions occur. For a reaction to occur: 1. Particles must meet/collide 2. They must collide with a certain minimum energy (activation energy) 3. Bonds must break (in the reactants) (*this requires energy*) 4. New bonds must form (products) (*this releases energy*)	*Endothermic*: heat gained from surroundings ΔH = positive. *Exothermic*: heat lost to surroundings ΔH = negative.

Chemistry: Elements, compounds and mixtures

Periodic table A way of grouping elements: a *Period* (horizontal row): outermost electron shell is filled as you move across; a *Group* (vertical column) contains elements with the same number of electrons in the outermost energy level, and hence similar properties.	Think about how common properties (e.g. m.p./b.p./mass/reactivity) change as you move down a Group or across a Period. Use the table as a tool to help you interpret the characteristics of all elements.

Elements
Made up of only one type of atom; 92 elements occur naturally and make millions of different substances.

Noble gases Group 0: The outermost shell is full, so these are unreactive: neither have a tendency to gain nor a tendency to lose electrons (or share them!)	What happens to common properties as you move down Group 0?

Alkali metals Group 1 (metals): React with non-metals to form ionic compounds. Outer shell contains a single electron. Reactions require outermost electron to be lost. If it is easy to lose the electron, the reactivity is higher. Significant reactions: Metal + water → metal hydroxide + hydrogen Metal + oxygen → metal oxide Metal oxide + water → metal hydroxide Metal + chlorine → metal chloride	*Reactivity*: K > Na > Li (increases down the Group) e.g. $2Na + 2H_2O \rightarrow 2NaOH + H_2$ e.g. $K + O_2 \rightarrow K_2O$ e.g. $K_2O + H_2O \rightarrow 2KOH$ e.g. $2Li + Cl_2 \rightarrow 2LiCl$
Halogens Group 7 (non-metals): Consist of diatomic molecules. Form molecular compounds with other non-metallic compounds. React with metals to form ionic compounds. Outer shell contains 7 electrons. Reactions require an electron to be gained to complete the outer shell. The easier it is to gain, the more reactive.	*Reactivity*: F > Cl > Br (decreases down the Group): this can affect displacement reactions e.g. $Cl_2 + 2KBr \rightarrow Br_2 + 2KCl$
Transition metals Have high m.p., high b.p.; are hard and strong; form coloured compounds. They are fairly unreactive with water; exhibit catalytic properties.	Compare with alkali "metals".
Compounds generally Compounds are chemically bonded. Ionic compounds form giant ionic lattices with high m.p.s and high b.p.s, usually dissolve in water. In the solid state, do not conduct electricity (ions are fixed), but may do so when molten/aqueous.	CO_2 is a compound of carbon and oxygen.
Mixtures Mixtures can be separated easily – the component parts have not reacted and are not chemically bonded.	Air is a mixture of various gases.
Separation generally Separation can occur due to differences in physical properties of substances in mixtures.	*Examples of separation*: Filtration, chromatography, fractional distillation.
Filtration The method of separating mixtures of insoluble solids and liquids.	
Chromatography Used to separate mixtures of solutes in a solution.	

Chemistry: Obtaining and using materials

Hydrocarbons
Compounds made up of carbon and hydrogen only. Many present in crude oil, can be separated into fractions by fractional distillation.

Plastics/polymers
Polymerisation: monomers join to form polymers.

Metals: Generally
Metals form giant structures which conduct electricity, are malleable and ductile.

Electrolysis	
The process where a molten or aqueous substance is decomposed after an electric current is passed through it. *During electrolysis*: Cations gain electrons at the cathode (gain of electrons = reduction) Cathode = negative electrode (attracts cations) Anode = positive electrode (attract anions) Anions lose electrons at the anode (oxidation) When molten compounds are electrolysed: the metal is deposited at the cathode; the non-metal is deposited at the anode. When aqueous salts are electrolysed, one must remember the hydrogen and oxygen present in the water: 1. If the metal is unreactive (below H_2 in the reactivity series), the metal is deposited (otherwise hydrogen is liberated from the water). 2. If the non-metal is from Group 7, this is liberated; otherwise oxygen is liberated.	• NaCl (molten) At cathode: $Na^+ + e^- \rightarrow Na$ At anode: $2Cl^- \rightarrow Cl_2 + 2e^-$ • KI(aq) At cathode: $2H^+ + 2e^- \rightarrow H_2$ (K is more reactive than H_2) At anode: $2I + I_2 \rightarrow 2e^-$ (Group 7) • $CuSO_4$(aq) At cathode: $Cu^{2+} + 2e^- \rightarrow Cu$ (since Cu is less reactive than H_2) At anode: $4OH \rightarrow O_2 + 2H_2O$ $+ 4e^-$

Nitrogenous fertilisers	
Ammonia is produced by the Haber process. Since ammonia is a base, it reacts with acids to form salts. Ammonium nitrate is a nitrogen fertiliser.	Ammonia + nitric acid → ammonium nitrate

Chemistry: Solids, liquids, gases

Changes of state	
Condensation: Gas → liquid Sublimation: Solid → gas	CO_2 commonly sublimes

Melting/boiling points	
Melting point: Temperature at which a solid → liquid (or liquid → solid). *Boiling point*: Temperature at which Liquid → gas; varies with pressure.	The higher the pressure, the higher the b.p. (impurities also increase b.p. and lower m.p.)

Density	
The amount of space taken up by a substance. If more of a substance is concentrated into a smaller area, the greater the density.	Density = mass/volume (kg/m^3 or g/cm^3)

Mathematics

Mathematics: Equations inequalities and functions

Equations and inequalities: General points

There are two ways equations or inequalities can be represented:

- as written equations or inequalities
- as graphs.

The best way to see how an equation/inequality works is to think of it in graphical form (sketch it out).
For *any* equation:

- the shape of the graph is determined by the function.
- substitute 0 for y to find where the graph crosses the x-axis (i.e. $y = 0$).
- substitute 0 for x to find where it crosses the y-axis (i.e. $x = 0$).

An equation or inequality is simply a "rule" that tells you how one variable relates to another. The graph is a diagram of this "rule" in action, using real values.

Linear equations

Generic form:

$$y = Ax + C$$

A: gradient of graph (change in y/change in x) (if A is negative, the gradient is negative).
C: y-intercept.

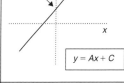

Quadratic equations

Definition: Any function where the highest power is a square.
Generic form:

$$y = x^2 + Bx + C$$

When factorised:

$$y = (x+P)(x+Q)$$

The "roots" of the equation are the values of x when $y = 0$ (the x-axis).
   In this case $-P$ and $-Q$
   P and Q *multiply* to give C and *add* to give B

Example 1:
For a quadratic equation, when $y = 0$, $x = +1$ and -3. What is the equation?

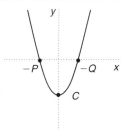

At the x-axis, $y = 0$, therefore:
$(x + P)(x + Q) = 0$
$x + P = 0, x = -P$
$x + Q = 0, x = -Q$

Answer: The roots of this equation are $+1$ and -3. Therefore: $y = (x + 3)(x - 1)$ *Opening out the brackets gives.* $y = x^2 + 2x - 3$ *Example 2:* The roots of a quadratic equation add up to 4 and multiply to 21. What is the equation? *Answer:* If we call the roots "p" and "q": we know that: $p + q = 4$ *and* $pq = 21$. In factorised form the equation must be: $y = (x - p)(x - q)$ open out the brackets: $y = x^2 - px - qx + pq$ $\qquad\qquad\qquad y = x^2 - x(p + q) + pq$ $\qquad\qquad\qquad y = x^2 - 4x + 21$	Tip When the roots of an equation are equal e.g. $y = (x + a)(x + a)$ i.e. $y = (x + a)^2$, this always opens out to give: $y = x^2 + a^2 + 2ax$
Quadratic inequalities *Example* Which values of x satisfy the inequality: $x^2 < 3x + 10$ *Answer:* Rearrange: $x^2 - 3x - 10 < 0$ if $x^2 = 3x + 10$ $x^2 - 3x - 10 = 0$ $(x + 2)(x - 5) = 0$ so the roots are -2 and 5 and the graph would look roughly like this: 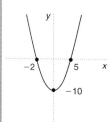 It is obvious from this that $x^2 - 3x - 10$ is less than 0 between -2 and 5, so the values of x satisfying this are: $-2 < x < 5$ (i.e. -1, 0, 1, 2, 3, 4) Common pitfall: when calculating the inequality: $(x + 2)(x - 5) < 0$ $x - 5 < 0, x = 5$ is correct; $x + 2 < 0$ is *not* correct!	*General approach:* 1. Solve as if it were an equation 2. Sketch the graph (very roughly!) 3. Then work out which values satisfy the inequality A quick-sketch graph is an easy way to solve an inequality. In general dividing an inequality by $(x - a)$ causes the sign to change, so the solution is: $x - 5 < 0, x < 5$ $x + 2 > 0, x > -2$ Inequalities do *not* always behave the same as equations.
Rearranging equations Equations are often represented in "jumbled form" e.g. $\dfrac{2y + y^2}{x} = 5$	These methods can be used for any algebraic fractions, usually one is quicker than the other, depending on the factors involved.

This requires rearrangement of the equation to make one variable the "subject".

Example: Make *a* the subject of the following equation and solve for *m*:

$$\frac{1}{a + 2} + \frac{a + 2}{4} = \frac{1}{m}$$

Answer: by multiplying both sides by a common factor, $(a + 2)$

$$1 + \frac{(a + 2)^2}{4} = \frac{1(a + 2)}{m}$$

so,

$$\frac{4 + (a + 2)^2}{4} = \frac{(a + 2)}{m}$$

$$m = \frac{4(a + 2)}{4 + (a + 2)^2}$$

or, another method: by finding a common denominator [the common denominator here is $4(a + 2)$], so multiply the first fraction, top and bottom by 4 and the second fraction, top and bottom by $(a + 2)$.

$$\frac{4 + (a + 2)^2}{4(a + 2)} = \frac{1}{m} \quad \rightarrow \quad m = \frac{4(a + 2)}{4 + (a + 2)^2}$$

Common pitfall:
Note that

$$1 + \frac{(a + 2)^2}{4} = \frac{1(a + 2)}{m}$$

cannot be directly transformed to:

$$1 + \frac{4}{(a + 2)^2} = \frac{m}{1(a + 2)}$$

A common denominator for any fraction can be found by multiplying the denominators together.

Trigonometric functions

The sin and cos functions are waves that repeat every 360°. Knowing the curves allows you to calculate all the possible values over a certain range. The following rules are worth remembering (as they make routine calculations quicker, but you can always derive this information from the curves themselves).

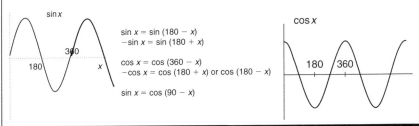

$\sin x = \sin (180 - x)$
$-\sin x = \sin (180 + x)$

$\cos x = \cos (360 - x)$
$-\cos x = \cos (180 + x)$ or $\cos (180 - x)$

$\sin x = \cos (90 - x)$

Mathematics: Numbers and the number system

Roots and surds

Numbers in the form "$\sqrt{x}$" can be treated just like any other number, with the additional rule that: $(\sqrt{x})^2 = x$.

You may be asked to use surds applied to a problem that requires additional skills from other parts of the syllabus.

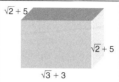

Example: A cuboid has dimensions $\sqrt{2} + 5$, $\sqrt{2} + 5$, $\sqrt{3} + 3$.

What is its surface area?

Remember, the rules applying to algebraic quadratic equations also apply here (or to any number!)

Answer: *2 squares and 4 rectangular surfaces*

$2(\sqrt{2} + 5)^2 + 4(\sqrt{2} + 5)(\sqrt{3} + 3)$

$2(2 + 25 + 10\sqrt{2}) + 4(\sqrt{2}\sqrt{3} + 3\sqrt{2} + 5\sqrt{3} + 15)$

simplifies to:

$114 + 32\sqrt{2} + 20\sqrt{3} + 4\sqrt{2}\sqrt{3}$

Powers and standard form

Standard form is a way of displaying a number in terms of a power of 10 in the form of $a \times 10^b$ where $1 \leq a < 10$.

Basic rules of powers:

$A^n \times A^n = A^{n+n}$

$$\frac{A^n}{A^n} = A^{n-n}$$

$(A^n)^n = A^{n \times n}$

$A^0 = 1$

$10^n = 10 \times 10 \times 10 \times \ldots$ [n times], or 1 with "n" zeroes after it

$10^{-n} = 1/10^n$

Exercise:

If planet A is a distance of 2.34×10^{18} miles from the centre of planet B and planet A orbits around B once every 850 days, what is the speed of planet A? (express your answer in miles/hour as standard form).

Answer: Speed of planet = distance/time

Distance of orbit = $(2\pi \times 2.34 \times 10^{18})$miles

Time of orbit = $(850 \times 24) = 20,400 = 2.04 \times 10^4$ hours

Speed = $(2\pi \times 2.34 \times 10^{18})/2.04 \times 10^4$

= 7.2×10^{14} miles/hour

Tip: It is easiest to group the powers of 10 and calculate them separately (in this case, $10^{18}/10^4 = 10^{14}$).

Mathematics: Interpreting data

Probability

In probability there are two main rules to be aware of:

- Probability of A *and* B = $P(A) \times P(B)$
- Probability of A *or* B = $P(A) + P(B)$

However, in addition to the probabilities of independent events, it is still important to consider *all* the possible *combinations* of events.

Example:

A bag contains 8 red, 12 yellow, 5 green and 5 blue balls. I pick out 3 balls at random, without looking inside. What is the probability that I will pick up at least 2 red balls?

$P(A)$, $P(B)$ – refer to the *independent* probabilities of those events occurring.

The answer to this example is not simply $(8/30 \times 8/30) + (8/30 \times 8/30 \times 8/30)$ because:

- the probability of each independent event *changes* as you remove balls from the bag
- not picking the red ball itself has a probability that needs to be accounted for
- the 2 red balls can be picked out in 3 *different combinations* of ways!

Answer: If R is the probability of picking a red, and NR is the probability of not.
We want the probability of 2 red balls:
$(R \times R \times NR) + (R \times NR \times R) + (NR \times R \times R)$
or 3 red balls: $(R \times R \times R)$

$= (8/30 \times 7/29 \times 22/28) + (8/30 \times 22/29 \times 7/28)$
$+ (22/30 \times 8/29 \times 7/28) + (8/30 \times 7/29 \times 6/28)$
$= 3 \times (8/30 \times 7/29 \times 22/28) + (8/30 \times 7/29 \times 6/28)$
$= 0.15 + 0.014$
$= 0.164$

Mathematics: Geometry and trigonometry

Angle properties of shapes
Triangles – all angles add up to $180°$

– isosceles – 2 angles and opposite sides equal
– equilateral – all angles and all sides equal
– right angled triangle: one $90°$ angle, with longest side opposite.

Quadrilaterals (including squares and rectangles) – all angles add up to $360°$

– Parallelograms – opposite sides are parallel and equal in length.
– Rhombus = parallelogram with all 4 sides equal. The diagonals of a rhombus are perpendicular to each other.
– Trapezium = 2 parallel sides.

Angles of any shape with "n" sides add up to $180n - 360$.
A regular polygon is one where all sides are the same length.

Angles at parallel lines:

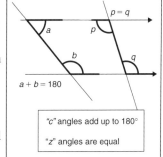

$a + b = 180$

"c" angles add up to $180°$

"z" angles are equal

Pythagoras' theorem
Apply only to right angled triangles

$\sin \theta = O/H$
$\cos \theta = A/H$
$\tan \theta = O/A$

"S.O.H - C.A.H - T.O.A"

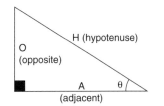

H (hypotenuse)
O (opposite)
A (adjacent)

Sine rule and cosine rule
For *any* triangle
Sine rule: Cosine rule:

$$\frac{a}{SinA} = \frac{b}{SinB} = \frac{c}{SinC}$$

$$a^2 = b^2 + c^2 - 2bcCosA$$

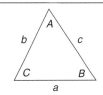

Circles: Generally

Area of circle = πr^2; Circumference = $2\pi r$

Area of sector = $\theta/360 \times \pi r^2$

Perimeter of sector = $(\theta/360 \times 2\pi r) + 2r$

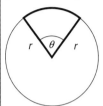

Circles: lines in circles

Intersecting chords.

The product of the distances from the circumference to the intersection point of each chord is equal. (This is also true for intersections outside the circumference.)

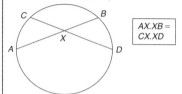

$AX.XB = CX.XD$

Circles: Angles in circles

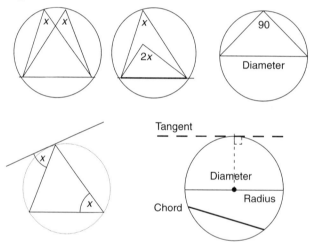

Triangles within circles:

- *From any chord*: the angle opposite the chord of any triangle that can be made with the circumference will be equal; if the triangle is made at the centre of the circle, the angle will be twice that of a triangle made at the circumference.
- *From the diameter*: the angle opposite the diameter of the triangle is 90°.
- *Alternate segment theorem*: the angle opposite the angle formed by a vector and vertex of a triangle are equal.

A tangent makes a right angle with the radius.

Physics

Physics: Forces and motion

Speed

Speed = rate of motion, measured in metres per second (m/s or ms^{-1}); the greater the speed the faster the body.

The speed of a body in everyday life is hardly ever constant: it changes from moment to moment (just think about driving a car). This is instantaneous speed – the speed of a body at any given instant – it is difficult to measure and unhelpful.

A more helpful measurement is average speed; the speed derived from taking the whole distance travelled and the time taken.

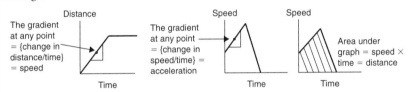

The gradient at any point = {change in distance/time} = speed

The gradient at any point = {change in speed/time} = acceleration

Area under graph = speed × time = distance

Speed is always positive (as distance covered can never be negative)

Acceleration

The rate of change of a body's speed is acceleration.

Acceleration can be negative (because the change of speed can be negative).

If the change in speed is negative it is known as negative acceleration or deceleration.

As long as acceleration is positive, speed is increasing.

$$\text{Acceleration} = \frac{\text{Change in Speed}}{\text{Time taken for change}}$$

SI units = m/s^2 or ms^{-2}

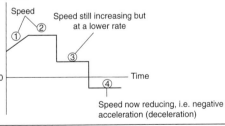

Speed still increasing but at a lower rate

Speed now reducing, i.e. negative acceleration (deceleration)

Forces generally

Force is measured in newtons (N).

Force always causes a body to accelerate or decelerate: an object will remain in a position of rest or keep moving at constant speed unless acted on by a net force. Making a body move from rest or changing its current speed both involve acceleration or deceleration.

Force = mass × acceleration ($F = ma$).

But this implies that a body can continue to move forever with a constant speed without any force acting on it!

This is true in a vacuum without any friction. In real life, there is always a force acting on a body to bring it to rest whenever it is in motion (drag forces).

Forces occur in pairs: When body A acts on body B with a force, body B acts on body A with the same force in an opposite direction.

There are different types of forces – non contact forces – due to force fields, e.g. electrostatic forces due to electric fields; and contact forces, e.g. push and pull forces.

> The greater the force acting on a given mass, the greater the acceleration.

Implications

Every body at rest or moving in a straight line at a constant speed *does not* have a net force acting on it.

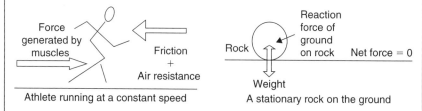

Athlete running at a constant speed

A stationary rock on the ground

In both cases Net force = 0 as there is no acceleration

Combining forces

There is usually more than one force acting on an object. The way the object behaves is a result of the combination of all the forces.

When all the forces acting on a body are combined – we get the *net force* acting on a body.

A free body diagram shows all the forces acting on an object thus helping us understand its behaviour (see above).

Weight and mass

Mass is the way we measure the quantity of matter in an object. It is measured in kilograms (kg). The greater the mass of an object, the greater the quantity of matter it contains. Mass is always there wherever you go in the universe and it is independent of gravity.

Weight is a force. The weight of an object is the force acting on it due to gravity. Without gravity there can be *no* weight.

As it is a force weight is measured in newtons (N).

In space where gravity is negligible – objects are weightless (they feel as light as a feather) but they still have mass.

The weight of an object depends on its mass, the greater the mass, the greater the gravitational pull, so the greater the weight.

Inertia is the reluctance of a body to any change to its state of rest or motion of constant speed, i.e. the tendency of a body to resist the effect of force.

Inertia depends on mass: the greater the mass of an object the greater the inertia.

Inertia is a body's reluctance to relinquish its state of stability (a body is stable when it is at rest or moving at a constant speed)

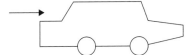

- To overcome inertia you need *force*
- Therefore a force always causes a body to move from rest or change its speed
- In other words, a net force always causes acceleration

Weight $=$ mass $\times$ g
What is g?
(Hint: $F = ma$)

Gravity

Every body attracts every other body in the universe by a force – gravity – which is a non-contact force.

Every object on earth (including humans) is attracted to the earth by this force of gravity and these objects in turn attract the earth by the same force (remember forces occur in pairs).

The force of gravity gives objects their weight and makes objects accelerate when they are in free fall.

The force of gravity acting on an object is its weight $F =$ weight (W)

The earth has a pulling force on every object around it because of its gravitational field

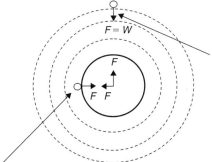

This force (like all forces) causes the body to accelerate when in free fall. This acceleration is known as *g* (acceleration due to gravity)

This force is still acting when the body is on the ground, but the body does not accelerate any more because this force is counter balanced by a contact force from the ground acting on the body as well. *Note* that each object also attracts the earth with a force equal to its weight but the earth doesn't move because it is so *massive*.

Friction and air resistance

Drag forces: Forces in the environment which act to resist motion. There are two main types – friction and air resistance.

Drag forces only act when a body is in motion, they do not act when a body is at rest. The faster the body attempts to move the stronger the drag forces act; they do not stop acting till the body comes back to rest.

Friction is the force that acts to resist motion of an object on the ground (or on any other surface for that matter). It is due to the fact that virtually all surfaces are uneven.

Air resistance is the force that acts on a body moving through the air as a result of the air particles bombarding the front surface of the object.

In real life we try to minimise drag forces in order to reduce the amount of time and energy wasted on overcoming them.

Friction: The intrinsic roughness of surfaces serves to oppose motion between surfaces in any direction.

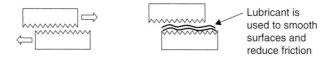

Lubricant is used to smooth surfaces and reduce friction

Air resistance: Caused by the action of air molecules on the moving object.

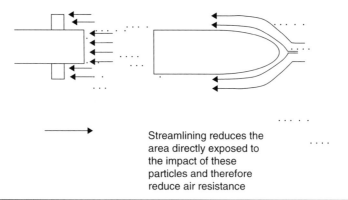

Streamlining reduces the area directly exposed to the impact of these particles and therefore reduce air resistance

Moments

We have seen that when the sum of forces acting on a body is zero, the body is stable or in equilibrium. But this is not the only requirement for equilibrium. Although the forces might not be able to make a body move from place to place, they might still be able to make the body rotate about a point (like a seesaw).

Such a turning force is called a moment.

So to be in equilibrium a body must have a net force of zero and also a net moment of zero.

The moment of a force increases if the force increases or if the distance from the pivot also increases.

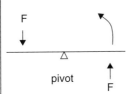

Moment = Perpendicular force × Distance from pivot

The net force on the body is 0 but the forces cause the body to rotate in an anticlockwise direction.

pivot

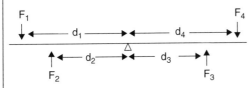

Net moments acting on rod
= Anticlockwise moments −
  Clockwise moments
= $(F_1 d_1 + F_3 d_3) - (F_2 d_2 + F_4 d_4)$
= If answer is *positive*
= Net moment is *anticlockwise*

If answer is 0 = No net moment
If answer is *negative* = Net moment is *clockwise*

Pressure

Pressure is force per unit area. It is measured in N/m^2 or Pascals.

Pressure can be increased by increasing the force or by reducing the area on which it acts.

Pressure is a way of determining what the impact of the force will be. A force over a large area is "dilute" and so will have a lower impact than the same force over a small area – which is more "concentrated" and thus will have a greater impact.

Fluid pressure is the same in all directions and can be transmitted from one part of the fluid body to another.

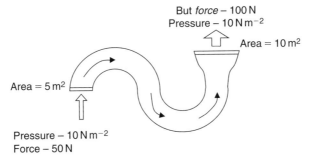

But *force* – 100 N
Pressure – 10 N m^{-2}
Area = 10 m^2

Area = 5 m^2

Pressure – 10 N m^{-2}
Force – 50 N

The pressure exerted at one end is the same as that which arrives at the other end. Fluid is used to transmit pressures and *increase* forces.

Floating and sinking

The density of an object is the mass per unit volume.

We know that some objects will float in a fluid while others will sink depending on their density.

Two principles determine the behaviour of objects in fluids.

Archimedes' Principle – an object immersed in a fluid will displace a *volume* of fluid equal to the volume of the object beneath the surface of the fluid. (This makes sense as two things cannot occupy the same space.) Principle of floatation – a floating object always displaces a *weight* of fluid equal to its own weight.

Implications:

When you lower an object in water for example, it will begin sinking (and as it does so displaces more and more water) until it has displaced an amount of water equal to its weight. And at that point it will stop sinking – and begin to float.

If the object becomes totally immersed and the amount of water displaced is not yet equal to its weight, it means it will sink as it cannot displace any more fluid (it is totally immersed).

It means that for an object to float it must be able to displace its weight in fluid before it becomes totally immersed. But since the volume of fluid displaced at that point will be less than the objects' volume, the object must be less dense than the fluid to be able to float.

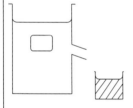

- Volume of immersed object is equal to volume of displaced fluid.
- Their weights are not necessary equal.

Object Floating

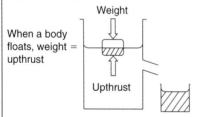

When a body floats, weight = upthrust

- Volume of part of object immersed = volume of fluid displaced.
- Weight of fluid displaced = weight of fluid.

The relative densities of the object and the fluid determine the proportion of the object beneath the fluid surface.

When an object is afloat, it is at rest (at least in the vertical direction) so must have a net force of zero.

This means the water is pushing up on it with a force equal to its weight.

This force is known as upthrust.

Every body in water experiences upthrust and the upthrust is equal to the weight of fluid displaced.

Physics: Energy

Energy generally
Energy is the ability to do work.

We cannot see energy but we can see the effect of energy when work is done.

Energy cannot be created or destroyed. The total amount of energy in the universe is constant.

When we "lose" energy by dissipating it, it has not been destroyed but has merely been transformed to another type of energy usually including heat.

There are different forms of energy, e.g. chemical, mechanical, electric, thermal.

There are various sources of energy – An important source of energy is the Sun.

Energy transformation and storage
Energy can be transformed from one form to another.

When energy is transformed, work is done and this is when we see the effect of energy.

Work done = Energy transferred = Joules.

Whenever energy is transformed (i.e. whenever work is done), some of it is lost as heat.

Energy transformed = New energy + Energy lost as heat.

Work done may be in various forms – electrical, chemical, mechanical, etc.

Mechanical work is only ever done when a force moves an object. If the force fails to move the object, work has not been done.

Mechanical work done = Force × distance

Energy can also be stored in the various forms in which it occurs. When energy is stored it is known as potential energy, e.g. chemical potential energy in the food we eat.

Chemical bonds are the way chemical energy is stored while force fields can also help to store energy, e.g. gravitational potential energy.

Kinetic and potential energy
Two important forms of energy are kinetic and potential energy.

Kinetic energy is the energy of motion. An object only has kinetic energy when it is in motion.

Kinetic energy = ½ mass × velocity^2
Kinetic energy = $\frac{1}{2}mv^2$

Potential energy is stored energy. An object has potential energy when work is done on the object for example moving it up a hill.

Gravitational potential energy = Force × distance
Weight × height
Mass × g × height

Work and power	SI Units
Power and work are not the same thing.	Energy = Joules (J)
Power is the rate of doing work. If two people do the same amount of work but one does it faster than the other then the faster person has more power.	Work = Joules (J) Power = Watts (W)
Power = Work done/time taken	
Since there are different types of work, there are also different types of power.	

Temperature and heat

Heat or thermal energy is a very common form of energy; it is always produced when energy is transformed from one form to another.

When an object acquires heat energy its particles move faster.

Temperature is a measure of this kinetic energy possessed by the particles of an object.

So heat energy causes objects to change their temperature as it changes the average kinetic energy of their particles.

The greater the heat energy of a liquid, the greater the kinetic energy of its particles.

The greater the average energy of the particles of a liquid the greater the number of particles that are able to escape from the surface.

This escape from the surface of a liquid is called evaporation.

Evaporation is more frequent at higher temperatures.

Conduction, convection, radiation

There are three main methods of heat transfer:

Conduction: Heat is transferred from one particle to the next until it reaches the destination. This is the method of transfer in solids as the particles in solids cannot move very far. Any material that can transfer heat in this way is called a conductor.

Convection: The particles actually move and so carry the heat energy with them wherever they go. The particles have to be very loosely attracted and so be able to move quite freely. Therefore it is common in liquids and gases.

Radiation: This is the way heat is transferred in a vacuum. It does not need a medium. This is the way heat is transferred in outer space.

Physics: Electricity and magnetism

Circuits generally

A circuit is a closed loop of a conductor around which current can flow.

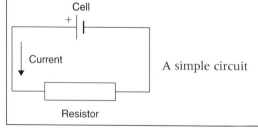

A simple circuit

Series, parallel circuits

Circuit components can be connected in series (one after the other) or in parallel (alongside each other).

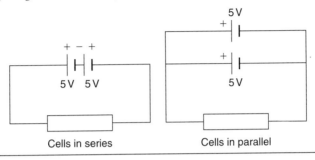

Cells in series   Cells in parallel

Voltage

Also known as electromotive force (e.m.f) or potential difference (p.d.), it is the energy given to each unit of charge by a cell. The source of voltage is the cell.

Voltage is the energy per charge. Therefore to find the total energy in a circuit = Voltage × total charge.

Since Power = energy/time.

Therefore Electric power = Voltage × total charge/time
= Voltage × current

Voltage is across a circuit which means to add the voltages of two cells in a circuit they must be arranged in series (one after the other).

A Battery is a collection of cells arranged in series.

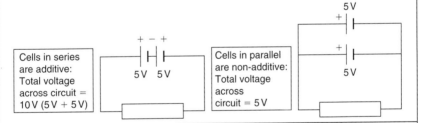

Electric current

It is the rate of flow of charged particles. Current flows through a circuit which means it must split at any points the circuit splits.

Conventional current is the flow of positive charges from positive to negative while in reality electricity is caused by the flow of electrons from the negative side of the battery all the way to the positive side.

Conventional current flows in the opposite direction to electrons.

Resistance

This is the opposition (resistance) to the flow of current.

In model circuits resistance is provided by a resistor. In real life, resistance is provided by the load(s) in the circuit.

Understanding resistors in parallel versus resistors in series.
Resistors in parallel:
Each resistor has the same voltage across it (the voltage of the Cell).

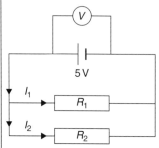

So for each resistor $V = I$ (the current flowing through it) $\times R$ (its own resistance).

To find the total current and the total resistance of the resistors in parallel:

Total I = Total V/Total R

But Total $I = I_1 + I_2$
So Total V/Total R = Total V/R_1 + Total V/R_2
Multiply both sides of the equation by (1/Total V)
So $1/\text{Total R} = 1/R_1 + 1/R_2$

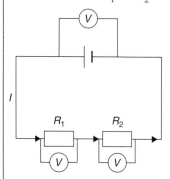

Resistors in series:
Since the voltage of the Cell is across the whole circuit, so the voltage across each resistor equals the total voltage. On the other hand, the circuit does not split at any point, so the same current flows through all resistors.
Since $V = IR$; the total voltage is split across each resistor in direction proportion to their resistances.

Total $V = V_1 + V_2$
$I(\text{Total } R) = IR_1 + IR_2$
Multiply both sides of the equation by $(1/I)$
Total $R = R_1 + R_2$

The same current flows through resistors when they are in series but they share the voltage in proportion to their resistances.

Electric charge	Charge = Current $\times$ time
Charge is the amount of electricity. The unit of charge is the coulomb (C). Since current is the rate of flow of charge, i.e. the amount of charge that flows every second, we can infer that to get the amount of charge, we need to know the current (the amount of charge per second) and the time (number of seconds) for which it has been flowing.	Current = Charge/time

Components in circuits

A circuit can be thought of as a closed loop of pipe with water flowing through it – the pipe is the circuit, the water is the electrical charge while the rate of flow of water is the current.

To keep the water flowing you need a pump which continually provides the water with energy to flow through the pipe – this is the Cell or Battery, the energy provided is the voltage.

You might also have a water wheel or something that provides some obstruction to the flow of the water – this is the resistor.

Ohm's law

Defines the relationship between voltage and current. Current= voltage/resistance

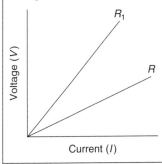

Graph of Ohm's Law
Ohm's law: Voltage is directly proportional to current.
So, resistance is the gradient of the voltage/ current graph.
Therefore $R_1 > R$.

Electrical quantities and symbols	SI units
Current = Charge [C]/time [t] Voltage = Current [I]×Resistance [R] Energy = Voltage [V]×Total charge [C] Power = Voltage [V]×Current [I]	Voltage= Volts (V) Charge= Coulombs (C) Resistance= Ohms (Ω) Energy = Joules (J) Power = Watts (W)

Fields and forces

A Force field is the imaginary area (field) around a body in which it exerts a force. It is the models we use to understand non-contact forces, i.e. forces acting at a distance.

There are different types of force fields: electric, magnetic and gravitational.

Electric fields: Like charges repel, unlike charges attract.

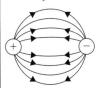

Magnetic fields: Like poles repel, while unlike poles attract. N=North Pole; S=South pole.

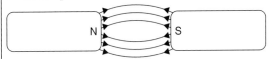

There is a strong interaction between electric and magnetic fields. Magnetic fields can cause charges to move, while electric fields can also cause magnets to move.

Gravitational fields: see previous.
You can store energy as a result of a field.

Electric motors and generators
Electric motors convert electric energy to mechanical energy. They do the opposite job to generators.

Generators or dynamos convert mechanical energy to electrical energy.

Transformers
Transformers convert an input voltage into a different output voltage.

Step-up transformer converts a small voltage into a large voltage.

Step-down transformer converts a large voltage into a small voltage.

$$\frac{\text{Turns on input coil}}{\text{Turns on output coil}} = \frac{\text{Input voltage}}{\text{Output}}$$

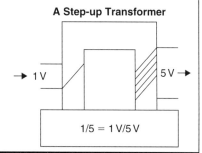

A Step-up Transformer

→ 1 V   5 V →

1/5 = 1 V/5 V

Physics: Waves

Wave characteristics generally
Waves are oscillations or vibrations. The vibrations happen in cycles with the wave moving away from the centre and then back through the centre in the opposite direction and back to the centre again. Then the cycle restarts.

There are different types of waves. Some require a substance through which to travel (mechanical waves) while others, interestingly, do not (electromagnetic waves).

Wave amplitude, frequency, speed and wavelength
A full vibration involves two movements in opposite directions (one cycle).

Frequency (f) is the number of cycles per second.

The amplitude of a wave is the maximum point of oscillation from the centre in either direction.

The length of one full cycle of a wave is the wavelength (λ).

The length of one cycle of a wave (λ)×the number of cycles in a second (f) = distance covered by the wave in a second (the speed).

Transverse waves
These wave oscillations occur in the up-and-down direction while the whole wave progresses in the left-to-right direction (or vice versa).

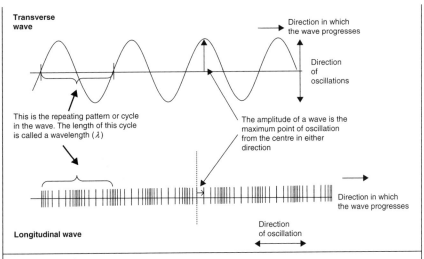

Longitudinal waves
In these waves the oscillations occur in the same direction as the progression of the whole wave.

Reflection, refraction and diffraction
Reflection happens when a wave bounces off an impenetrable surface. The wave is totally unchanged except that it changes direction.

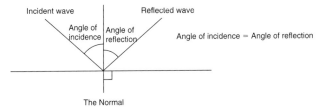

Refraction occurs when a wave moves from one medium into another medium and the speed changes. The direction of the wave may also change.

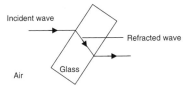

Diffraction occurs when a wave bends round the edge of an obstruction.

Electromagnetic spectrum
Disturbances which cause oscillations in electric and magnetic fields give rise to electromagnetic waves.

Since these fields are imaginary, these waves do not need any substance to be transmitted (unlike mechanical waves like sound waves).

Depending on the disturbance, the electromagnetic waves will have different wavelengths and frequencies.

All electromagnetic waves have the same speed – 300 million m/s – but different wavelengths.

Therefore they must have different frequencies as:

Wavelength $\times$ frequency = Speed

In order of increasing wavelength $\longrightarrow$

Gamma rays – X-rays – Ultraviolet – Visible light – Infrared – Microwaves – Radio waves

$\longleftarrow$ In order of decreasing frequency

Physics: Light

Light generally

Light, visible light that is, is a type of electromagnetic wave.

The Sun is the main source of visible light.

As it is an electromagnetic wave it does not need a medium for transmission.

It can move through a vacuum.

Properties of light generally

The main features of light are brightness and colour.

All types of light waves as well as all types of electromagnetic waves have the same *speed*. They differ in their frequencies and wavelengths.

$$\text{Speed of wave } (c) = \text{Frequency } (f) \times \text{wavelength } (\lambda)$$

Therefore visible light travels at 300 million m/s in a vacuum.

Reflection and refraction

As typical for waves, light undergo reflection and refraction according to the rules discussed previously.

Colour

Colour depends on the frequency of the light wave.

Visible light occurs in a whole range of frequencies and wavelengths called the visible spectrum.

The human eye interprets the different wavelengths as different colours.

Physics: Sound

Sound generally

Sound waves are longitudinal waves produced by disturbance to molecules (gases, liquids and solids).

Although sound is usually propagated in the air they can also be propagated through solids and liquids.

Sound travels at different speeds in different media – it travels fastest in solids, intermediate speeds in liquids and is slowest in gases.

Properties of sound: Generally

Sound has three main characteristics – loudness, pitch and quality

Loudness

The loudness of sound depends on the amplitude of the sound waves.

The greater the amplitude the louder the sound.

Pitch

The pitch of a sound depends on the frequency of the sound waves.

The higher the frequency the higher the pitch.

Humans are only able to hear frequencies between 20 Hz and 20,000 Hz. This is called the audible range.

Sound waves with frequencies just above the audible range are known as *ultrasound*. These cannot be heard by the human ear but are used in medicine for imaging of some internal organs.

Quality

Quality or timbre of sound is the pattern of frequencies that make up a sound.

Timbre is what gives a sound its uniqueness.

Most sounds you hear are not smooth cyclical tones you see in books including this one!

The waves are usually not so smooth and made up of sounds of different frequencies.

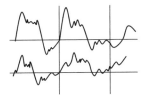 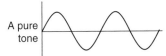

A pure tone

"Real" sounds (left) of broadly similar frequencies with different qualities.
The various peaks, notches and troughs imbue sounds with their uniqueness.
A pure tone (right) is a sound of one frequency only.

Physics: Radioactivity

Nuclear decay

Most nuclei form the stable core of atoms but some nuclei are unstable.

These are usually the unstable nuclei of the unstable isotopes of normally stable atoms – these isotopes are called radioisotopes.

When unstable nuclei break apart – it is called nuclear decay.

They are said to emit radioactivity.

There are three main kinds of radioactivity – alpha (α), beta (β) and gamma (γ).

An important effect of radiation of this sort is ionisation – the ability to knock off electrons in the outer shells of atoms as they whiz past them. This converts the atoms into ions (ionisation). This is an important cause of cancer as ionisation of atoms in DNA can cause them to behave abnormally.

Also because the radiation emitted is made up of such small particles, they are able to penetrate through substances, moving through the spaces found between atoms in matter. The smaller the radiation, the more the penetration.

Background radiation

We are all constantly exposed to radiation that comes from the naturally – occurring radioactive substances in the Earth and air all around and from space as well but also as a result of man-made radioactivity, mainly X-rays from medical use.

This is called background radiation.

It is minimal and so generally *not* harmful.

Alpha/beta/gamma radiation

Alpha (α) particles consist of two protons and two neutrons. Largest size, least penetrating but most ionising.

$$^{238}_{92}U \longrightarrow ^{234}_{90}Th + ^{4}_{2}\alpha$$

Beta (β) radiation consists of high energy electrons. Medium in size, penetration and ionising ability.

$$^{14}_{6}C \longrightarrow ^{14}_{7}N + ^{0}_{-1}e$$

Gamma (γ) radiation is part of electromagnetic spectrum. No size (it is a wave), most penetrating but least ionising.

$$^{60}_{26}Ni \longrightarrow ^{60}_{28}Ni$$

Activity

The activity of a radioactive material is a measure of how much radiation it produces, i.e. how radioactive it is.

This is the amount of radiation per unit time or the amount of decayed atoms per unit time.

The amount of a substance that has decayed is directly proportional to the amount of radiation that has been produced.

Half-life

Given a sample of radioactive material, it takes a certain time *t* for half of the material to decay, but then after another period of the same time *t*, only half of what was left has decayed.

It has a constant half-life. (The time it takes for half of a sample of radioactive material to decay is the half-life of the material.)

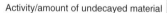
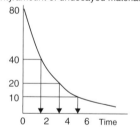

Activity/amount of undecayed material

This means the rate of decay of a radioactive substance is proportional to the number of undecayed nuclei at any particular time.

This must mean that the rate of decay reduces with time as the quantity of material reduces.

The rate of radioactive decay is exponential.

Exponential means the rate of decay reduces with time. First being quick then getting slower and slower.

Part C: Practice

1 The following table shows the nutritional composition of three different meals, A, B and C. The relative amount of a nutrient in each meal ranges from none (expressed as "0") to a large amount (expressed as "+++").

	Protein	Carbohydrate	Fat	Iron	Vitamin C	Vitamin D	Energy
Meal A	++	++	+	+	++	++	++
Meal B	+	+	+++	0	0	+	++
Meal C	++	+++	+	++	+	0	+++

Based on the information in the table select which of meal would be most appropriate for each of the individuals below (tick the appropriate box):

A Patient with diabetes   Meal A ☐   Meal B ☐   Meal C ☐
B Patient with rickets (brittle bones) Meal A ☐   Meal B ☐   Meal C ☐
C Patient with scurvy   Meal A ☐   Meal B ☐   Meal C ☐
D Pregnant woman   Meal A ☐   Meal B ☐   Meal C ☐
E Patient with Anaemia (low Hb)   Meal A ☐   Meal B ☐   Meal C ☐

2 Egested material is analysed for its composition to detect defects of chemical digestion in different parts of the digestive tract. The following table shows the nutritional composition of a sample of egested material from five patients on the same diet. The relative amount of a nutrient in each sample ranges from none (expressed as "0") to a large amount (expressed as "+++").

	Starch	Maltose	Glucose	Protein	Amino Acids	Fats	Emulsified fats
A	++	0	++	0	0	++	0
B	++	+	0	+	0	++	0
C	+	+	0	+	+	0	0
D	+	++	0	+	0	+	++
E	0	++	0	+++	0	+	0

Which of the above options best corresponds to a patient with a defect in:

(i)   The stomach?
(ii)   The duodenum?
(iii) The ileum?

3 Which of the following is compatible with the path of a molecule of glucose from the intestine to the vena cava?

A Villus → Liver capillary → Hepatic portal vein → Tissue fluid → Lymph fluid → Vena cava
B Villus → Hepatic portal vein → Liver cell → Hepatic vein → Vena cava
C Villus → Lacteal → Lymph fluid → Tissue fluid → Vena cava

D Lacteal → Lymph fluid → Hepatic vein → Vena cava
E Villus → Mesenteric vein → Vena cava

4 From the list (labelled **A–I**) below, choose the correct sequence of six events that would allow a red blood cell in an alveolar capillary in the lungs to enter the systemic circulation.

A Blood moves into left atrium
B Ventricles contract
C Blood enters the aorta
D Blood enters the pulmonary vein
E Blood leaves via the pulmonary artery
F Semilunar valves open
G Bicuspid valve opens
H Tricuspid valve opens
I Blood enters the ventricles

_____ → _____ → _____ → _____ → _____ → _____

5 An athlete undertakes a specialised training scheme at high altitude to improve his fitness. Which *one* of the following changes is most likely to improve his ability to undertake greater levels of activity at altitude?

A An increase in the concentration of haemoglobin in his blood
B An increase in the number of red blood cells in his blood
C An increase in the volume of each breath
D An increase in anaerobic respiration
E An increase in the oxygen requirement of his muscles

6 The family-tree shows the inheritance of disease X in a family (dark circles and squares represent presence of the disease).

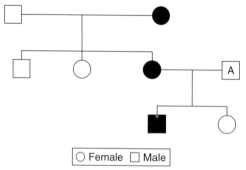

O Female □ Male

The disease is conveyed by means of defective alleles. If individual A has no defective alleles, which one of the following best describes the pattern of inheritance of this disease based on the information above?

A Autosomal dominant
B Autosomal recessive
C Co-dominant

D X-chromosome-linked recessive

E Y-chromosome-linked

7 The following is a timeline representing part of the menstrual cycle in a human.

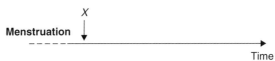

Which one of the following is the best order of events that may occur around and soon after point X.

A Corpus luteum dies

B Corpus luteum produces progesterone

C Fertilisation of ovum

D Implantation of zygote

E Oestrogen production

F Ovulation

G Shedding of womb lining

H Thickening of womb lining

(i) $e \to f \to b \to h \to c \to a \to g$ -

(ii) $f \to b \to h \to c \to d$

(iii) $f \to h \to c \to d \to b$ and e

(iv) $e \to f \to b \to c \to d$ -

(v) $f \to h \to a \to g$

8 Two mice, one with brown fur and one with white fur are bred, producing offspring as follows:

Brown fur: 25%; white fur: 25%; mottled (brown and white) fur: 25%; black fur: 25%

If two of the offspring with mottled fur are bred, what proportion of their offspring will also be mottled? _____%

9 The diagram below shows a hydroponics system for growing a plant. This is where nutrient solution replaces soil so that plant growers can carefully control the elements which the plant needs for optimal growth. The nutrient solution contains nitrogen (N), potassium (K) and phosphate (P).

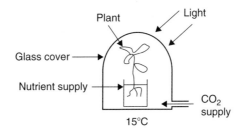

A plant grower wishes to test whether 10 ml calcium carbonate ($CaCO_3$) solution added to the nutrient solution improves plant growth. What would be the most suitable control nutrient solution for this experiment?

A N+P+K+10 ml distilled water
B N+P+K
C 10 ml $CaCO_3$ solution
D N+P+K+$CaCO_3$ solution at 25°C
E N+P+K+$CaCO_3$ solution at 15°C

10 The diagram below shows a schematic representation of energy flow through an ecosystem.

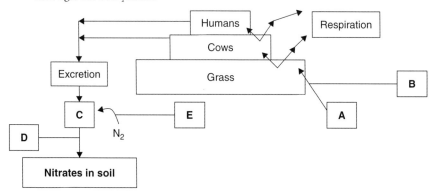

Choose an option (**A–E**) from the diagram to represent:

(i)   The process represented by the equation: $N_{2(g)} + 3H_{2(g)} \leftrightarrow 2NH_{3(g)}$
(ii) Nitrifying bacteria
(iii) The process for which chlorophyll is essential

11 In the red blood cell dihydroxyacetone phosphate is converted to glyceraldehyde 3-phosphate during glycolysis as shown below:

$$
\begin{array}{ccc}
CH_2OPO_3^{2-} & & H-C=O \\
| & & | \\
C=O & \rightarrow & H-C-OH \\
| & & | \\
CH_2OH & & CH_2OPO_3^{2-}
\end{array}
$$

This is an example of which one of the following chemical changes?

A Oxidation
B Isomerisation
C Reduction
D Thermal decomposition
E Dehydration

12 An element Z forms an ion Z^{3-}. How many protons are present in the nucleus of an atom of Z if the ion contains 51 electrons?

	Number of protons
A	48
B	49
C	50
D	51
E	54

13 Choose the correct word or term (labelled **A–J**) from the list below to match each numbered blank space (**i–vi**) in the following passage. No word or term is to be used more than once.

A atomic   **F** molecule(s)
B charge(s)   **G** neutron(s)
C electron(s)   **H** proton(s)
D isotope(s)   **I** radioactive
E mass   **J** toxic

Iron exists in several forms. The most abundant is iron-56. Iron-54 and even iron-58 exist, but these ......(i)...... are less abundant. All three elements mentioned above have the same ......(ii)...... number, but differ in ......(iii)...... number. Compared with iron-54 for example, iron-56 has two extra ......(iv)...... in the nucleus. The number of ......(v)...... and ......(vi)...... in all elements remain the same.

14 You are provided with an abbreviated periodic table below:

H																	
Li	Be											B	C	N	O	F	Ne
Na	Mg											Al	Si	P	S	Cl	Ar
K	Ca	Sc	Ti	V	Cr	Mn	Fe	Co	Ni	Cu	Zn	Ga	Ge	As	Se	Br	Kr
Rb	Sr											In	Sn	Sb	Te	I	Xe
Cs	Ba											Tl	Pb	Bi	Po	At	Rn

    (i)   neon (Ne)
    (ii)   fluorine (F)
    (iii)   potassium (K)
    (iv)   lithium (Li)
    (v)   nitrogen (N)
    (vi)   bromine (Br)
    (vii)   calcium (Ca)
   (viii) iron (Fe)

Can you correctly match the options (**A–E**) below with the correct elements listed above (**i–viii**)?

A Reacts with oxygen to form acidic oxides

B Belongs to the same Group as rubidium (Rb), but is less reactive, and has a higher melting point than sodium

C Belongs to the same Period as iron (Fe), and sinks as it reacts with water

D Belongs to the same Group as chlorine (Cl), but is less reactive

E Is a monatomic gas at room temperature and pressure

15 Balance the following equation:

$$pNO + qO_2 + rH_2O \rightarrow sHNO_3 + rNO$$

16 The diagram below shows the apparatus used for the electrolysis of aqueous sulphuric acid.

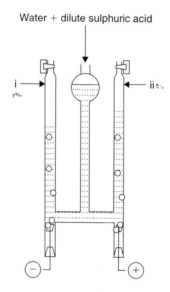

Water + dilute sulphuric acid

Match the correct use or property (labelled **A–D**) from the list below with the gaseous products (**i** or **ii**). If neither is applicable, choose option (**iii**). If both answers are applicable, choose option (**iv**). The answer options may be used once, more than once or not at all.

A reacts with nitrogen from air to produce ammonia ☐

B non-metal with low melting point ☐

C reacts with oxygen to form a toxic, poisonous gas ☐

D can be identified by the ability to relight a glowing splint ☐

17 The table below shows the physical properties of four compounds **i–iv**

	Melting point/K	Boiling point/K	Electrical conductivity in:		
			Solid state	Molten state	Aqueous state
i	371	1163	Yes	Yes	Yes
ii	831	1779	No	Yes	Insoluble
iii	14	20	No	No	Insoluble
iv	1028	1663	No	Yes	Yes

Which option (**A–E**) below shows the correct combination of the type of bonding present in the compounds listed **i–iv** above?

	i	ii	iii	iv
A	Giant metallic	Giant ionic	Small covalent	Giant ionic
B	Giant covalent	Giant metallic	Giant ionic	Small covalent
C	Giant metallic	Giant ionic	Small covalent	Giant covalent
D	Small covalent	Giant ionic	Giant covalent	Giant metallic
E	Giant metallic	Giant covalent	Giant ionic	Small covalent

18 What is the "specific latent energy of fusion" of a substance, if it takes a heat source of 20 kW power working for 20 minutes to totally melt 1000 kg of the substance all at the same temperature?

A 24 million J/g
B 24 thousand J/g
C 12 thousand J/g
D 12 million J/g
E 2 thousand J/g

19 A 30 g ball is brought to rest from a constant speed of 10 m/s in 5 seconds. What was the average force applied to the ball?

A 0.06 N
B 0.15 N
C 15 N
D 20 N
E 60 N

20 A resistor of 5 ohms has a current of 10 A running through it. What is the energy per unit charge dissipated in the resistor?
_____ J/C

21 Which of the following is least accurate?

A Sound waves are transverse waves
B Sound waves can have different wavelengths
C Sound waves are mechanical waves
D Not all sound waves are audible
E Sound waves can be transmitted in all directions from the point of origin

22 The graph of radioactive decay below was drawn by a student studying the behaviour of a radio-isotope for an assignment. All the data is accurate. What is the half-life of the radioisotope?_____ seconds.

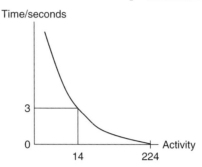

23 The model lever below has a movable bar balanced on a pivot. On one end is a 15 kg counterbalance while there is a mass M on the other end. The lever is in equilibrium. By how much and in what direction should the bar be moved on the pivot to have a total moment of 500 N/m? ($g = 10\,\text{m/s}^2$)

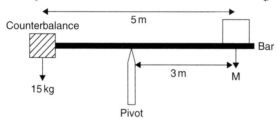

By_____ meters to the_____.

24 Rearrange the following to make x the subject:

$$\frac{(x + a)^2 + (x - a)^2}{2x} = \frac{1}{x}$$

A $x = \pm \sqrt{(1 - a^2)}$
B $x = \pm \sqrt{(-a^2)}$
C $x = \sqrt[3]{2}$
D $x = \pm \sqrt{(2/x)}$
E $x = 1/x - a^2$
F $x + 1/x = a^2$

25 Which of the following are correct simplifications of the equation:

$$2x + \frac{2}{x} = 8$$

A $(x - 2)(x - 6) = 0$
B $(x - 2)^2 = 3$

C $x^2 - 8x + 12 = 0$
D $2(x + 1)(x + 2) = 0$
E $2x = 0$

26 The sum of the roots of a quadratic equation are 0. What is the equation, assuming the roots are whole numbers?

A x^2+1
B x^2-2
C x^2+3
D x^2-4
E x^2+5

27 $\dfrac{4(x + a)}{2} - \dfrac{x + a}{4} = 2$

Which of the following would not satisfy the above equation?

A $x = a$
B $x > 3a$
B $x = -a$
D $x < a$

28 The diagram, which is not drawn to scale, shows two triangles sharing a common side, PQ, which is also the diameter of the circle as shown. If the diameter PQ is 10 cm and angles BQP = 25° and $x = 80°$, find the length of the side AQ (use the table below as required).

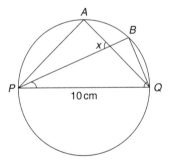

Not to Scale

x	25	30	35	40	45	50	55	60	65	70	75
sin x	0.42	0.5	0.57	0.64	0.71	0.77	0.82	0.87	0.91	0.94	0.97

29 Which of the following correctly expresses the perimeter of segment A?

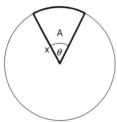

A $x\left(2 + \dfrac{\pi\theta}{180}\right)$

B $2x\left(1 + \dfrac{\theta}{360}\right)$

C $2x\left(1 + \dfrac{\pi\theta}{360}\right)$

D $2x(1 + \pi)$

30 Triangle A is a right-angled triangle. Find the length of a.

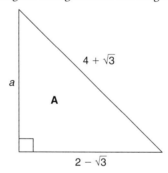

A $\sqrt{12}$
B $12(1+\sqrt{3})$
C $\sqrt{\{12(1+\sqrt{3})\}}$
D $26+4\sqrt{3}$
E $\sqrt{(26+4\sqrt{3})}$

31 In an office, 10% of workers have a hot breakfast and 20% have a hot lunch. What is the probability that a worker chosen at random will have at least one hot meal? (Assume breakfast and lunch are the only hot meals considered.)

A 26%
B 28%
C 30%
D 32%
E 34%

32 In a 3-ball lottery, three numbered balls are released from a chamber. The number of even-numbered balls in the chamber is twice the number of odd-numbered balls. What is the probability that at least 2 of the 3 released balls will be odd? Assume that there are 12 balls in the chamber and balls are released without replacement.

    A 78/330
    B 2/9
    C 2/27
    D 1/3
    E 4/27

33 Julie's mother bakes a cake which is normally a certain size. The amount of ingredients she uses normally is a. Julie's mother wants to bake a cake with a radius longer than normal by a factor r and with a height greater than normal by a factor h. What would be the amount of ingredients she would have to use?

    A $a (a + r)^2 (a + h)$
    B $a + (a + r^2) (a + h)$
    C $a (1 + r^2) (1 + h)$
    D $a (1 + r^2) (1 + h)^2$
    E ar^2h

CHAPTER 4

The Writing Task for the BMAT

Part A: First glance

What is Section 3 of the BMAT?

Section 3 of the BMAT is called The Writing Task. You have to choose one question to answer from a choice of 3. You have a time limit of 30 minutes and a space limit of a single side of an A4 page.

This is the subtlest part of the BMAT, assessing an intricate mesh of important skills. Unlike the previous two sections, the Writing Task does not only measure the end product of your thinking process but also the *process* itself: the way you choose, synthesise and communicate information.

Wherever you had to solve Critical Thinking questions previously, it was always about picking apart the argument. Now, in Section 3, you are writing the argument. You will score highly if you can make powerful arguments clearly and succinctly.

By now, having read and understood Chapter 2 on Critical Analysis, you should know how to recognise an argument. You should feel comfortable looking for the conclusion of an argument, spotting assumptions or thinking about ways to strengthen or weaken any part of it. As well as being used in the Critical Thinking component of BMAT Section 1, these skills are vitally important because they apply to Section 3 of the BMAT.

It is also the only part of the test over which you can exert some control: you have a choice of three questions, so you should choose carefully in order to produce your best answer possible. This is part of the test where you can *greatly* improve performance by practice.

Summary: Section 3 is about argument construction.

What *is not* Section 3 of the BMAT?

Sometimes Section 3 is called the "essay" section. This is fine as a shorthand for saying "BMAT Section 3: The Writing Task". But the BMAT "essay" is not the classic essay that you may have written once in English Literature or History class at school. You need to move away from the traditionally held view of how essays are written.

The most obvious difference is length. Essays are usually longer and the more you write the better you are perceived to be. The Writing Task is somewhat the opposite. After all, you are limited in space and time and so if you want to make several points you cannot afford to be uneconomical in your language. This is to encourage *thought* before committing pen to paper.

Secondly in a traditional essay, you usually have to write an introduction at the beginning and a conclusion at the end. The Writing Task (although a unified task) is still a response to several specific questions. You don't have to waste time introducing the subject and closing at the end – except it adds real *value* to your work. Otherwise jump straight in and finish when you do not have any more to say.

Thirdly, you have probably been told to write essays in continuous prose. The Writing Task asks you simply to communicate. If you find that bullet points, headings, short notes or diagrams help you make your point more clearly than continuous prose then you may do that. You are encouraged to do this as it communicates clearly your understanding.

Summary: The BMAT Writing Task is not your classical essay.

SCENARIO

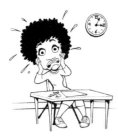 So, it's the big day. You've just done Sections 1 and 2. You're downhearted and tired. They've handed out Section 3 and you're told to begin. You turn the page and there are three questions staring back at you. You now have only 29 minutes 58 seconds left. What do you do?!

Option A – The gamble: You read through all the questions and see which one jumps out at you. Then you go for it.

Option B – The half-hearted approach: You read through all the questions and choose one randomly. You then begin to plan your answer in rough and you think you have enough to say so you go with that one and start to write.

You decide to go for Option A.

You get your head down and put pen to paper starting to write with the speed of a Japanese bullet train. "Oh, what a relief!" you think. Fifteen minutes into it and three-quarters of the way down the page you finally think you can come up for some air. But, oh my word, a quick glance at the question makes you realise that disaster has struck. You hadn't quite understood the question properly and so you have been answering the wrong question. What do you do now?!

"The Ostrich approach": pretend you haven't noticed and pretend that the examiner will understand and continue as before.

"Damage limitation": read through your answer from the beginning and start to cross out all irrelevant points whilst trying to squeeze in replacement answers between the lines.

"Honourable exit": in the remaining quarter of the page write a note to the examiner explaining what has happened, apologising and begging for her forgiveness and saying how you think you're not worthy to go to medical school and hope she has pity on you.

Part B: The approach

This section of the BMAT is difficult, without proper training. We will show you how to approach this and things to avoid:

1 Stay calm

This process should be done preferably before turning over the page for Section 3. Take time to calm yourself and focus on what is coming, not on what has gone. You will find no benefit in worrying about the previous two sections now (although feel free to dissect them at great length when you leave the exam room!). It is human nature to focus on things that you think went badly and forget the things that you completed well, so you will be muddying the waters with recall bias now anyway. It is difficult to gauge your performance, so don't (at least not now). Now is the time to maximise your overall BMAT score with a cracking Writing Task!

Bottom line: 30 minutes is not as short as you think: you have time.

2 Make a plan

Obviously the gambler's approach from the Scenario above is not the way we would recommend you go about answering Section 3 of the BMAT! But this is the way that most students, in our experience, go about answering the Writing Task. Why is this a bad strategy?

(a) How can you choose to answer one question on a gut instinct after a quick glance. Or, to put it another way, how can you dismiss the other questions so quickly? You need to stop and think about it. Many times the question you initially think you can answer the best is not actually the question you can answer the best!

(b) Most importantly: It is *impossible* to write an excellent answer without thinking and planning. It is as simple as that. This is a test of how you think – so think! This cannot be emphasised enough. You may even plan answers to more than one or all questions to see which one has the most material for the final answer.

How do I make a plan?

Using the schema below will guide you through the process of making a plan for any question.

READ AND UNDERSTAND THE QUESTION
⇓
QUESTION THE QUESTION (If necessary)
⇓
SELECT AND ORGANISE IDEAS
⇓
DEVELOP IDEAS

READ AND UNDERSTAND THE QUESTION: What does this mean?

Before you can answer the question, you need to read it and understand what is being asked. This sounds obvious but it is a vital skill. You should consider what *key words* are in the question. You must answer the questions being asked and the first step is identifying them. Understanding the question is especially important in the BMAT as you may be faced with difficultly-worded questions.

QUESTION THE QUESTION: What does this mean?

Many times the questions will be broad in scope, and may have multiple interpretations or many implications. Obviously in the time allotted you cannot cover everything. So feel free to define the limits of your question, whilst acknowledging that the question is complex.

SELECT AND ORGANISE IDEAS: What does this mean?

Questions in this section are usually broad in scope and the first thing being tested is your ability to select ideas: it is sometimes possible to write a whole book on many of the questions and you have only one A4 side and half an hour, so a good amount of *abstraction* – getting to the heart of the issue – is required. So before writing you need to think about the *main* ideas that make up your answer.

The ideas selected must then be organised to form a logical, consistent whole – you must understand the way your ideas link with each other and therefore place them in some coherent order which will make sense and flow smoothly in the final answer. Disorganised ideas betray a lack of understanding and thought. Make sure you answer all parts of the question in the right proportions (i.e. do not write half a page answering the first part of the question and leave only a few lines for your argument).

Your ideas and the order in which they should flow form the backbone of your answer. You should endeavour to deal with each idea separately and make this clear to the reader. In other words your answer should have structure – for instance, part (a) should be separate from part (b) and part (1) separate from part (2) and this should be obvious to the reader. You can do this by using bullet points, subheadings or mere spaces. Making it legible (able to be read) and presentable (pleasing on the eye) will help the marker award you the score you deserve.

DEVELOP IDEAS: What does this mean?

Once you have your main points in some logical structure and understand the overall picture it may be necessary to expand or develop some of your main points. For example, a few sentences to explain what you mean *convincingly*, or some examples to drive home your point will help produce a piece of clearly written text.

Bottom line: Before writing your answer in best you must make a plan.

Part C: Practice

The following section illustrates the points made so far. We have used actual (unedited) sample student essays of varying standard, with marker's comments and scores to show common pitfalls as well as shining examples. After reading these there is a section where you are allowed to comment and score some essays for yourself. Make sure you try each question for yourself first before looking at the answers and comments.

Before we give you the question, we thought that we needed to emphasise once more *the single most important factor in determining how well your answer is scored*: *planning*.

How much time should I spend on planning?

Well, you know how long you are allowed – 30 minutes.

How long does it take you, at maximum writing speed, to fill 1 side of A4? Maybe 10–15 minutes? Your writing speed as well as your thinking speed should determine this. Practice is also necessary to determine this (and possibly increase your speed!) But you don't HAVE to fill the whole side. If you can be succinct all the better! The time you didn't spend on writing will have been better spent thinking about the best way to communicate your ideas.

Now, try this question:

Example question 1

People should take some responsibility for their own health: the treatment of self-inflicted diseases should not be the responsibility of doctors in the NHS.

Write a unified essay in which you address the following:

1 Explain what you think this statement means.
2 What do you think the author had in mind by the term "self-inflicted diseases"?
3 Advance an argument against the statement above, i.e. "the treatment of self-inflicted diseases should be the responsibility of doctors in the NHS".

Try this answer for yourself, *before* going any further. See what you come up with (bearing in mind the guidelines above) and compare your essay with the samples below.

Scoring Essays

A quick word on how the Writing Task is scored. In the BMAT, two markers score each essay. If they give different scores, you can get an average of those scores (e.g. marker 1 scores you 6; marker 2 scores you 9; your average score is 7.5). Occasionally there is discrepancy by more than one scoring band (e.g. marker 1 scores you 6; marker 2 scores you 12); in this case the answer is marked by a third marker and a consensus is reached.
The criteria used are summarised below:

Score 0 = completely off-topic or missing.
Score 3 = A slight attempt at answering the question asked.
Score 6 = A fair attempt identified. Generally OK.
Score 9 = A good attempt has been made covering all areas asked, sound
and rational overall.
Score 12 = Same as for 9, but with a more impressive logic or command of
language.
Score 15 = Same as for 12, but leaving you saying "I could not have put it
better myself."

Sample Answers

Marker's Overview
For this question, as for any other, follow the schema as recommended above. You need to read the statement in bold and the three questions carefully.

Question 1 is simply asking what the statement means. You should use this
question to define your terms of reference. It can probably be answered
in a few sentences.
Question 2 is similar to question 1 so you need to realise this before you
start writing so that you do not end up repeating yourself. Making a
plan would solve this. You need to give a more specific definition here to
explain "self-inflicted diseases". Some examples may add value to your
answer.
Question 3 is asking you to make a counterargument against the statement
in bold. You are provided with the conclusion of the argument, and you
have to make valid reasons to support this.

SAMPLE STUDENT ESSAY 1

Civilisation should not take the NHS for granted. People should be looking after themselves instead of letting themselves go and then relying on the NHS for an organ donation or immediate surgery etc. People should attempt to live a healthy lifestyle and control their needs, for example do appropriate exercise, etc. Doctors should not need to treat patients who suffer from diseases that are self-inflicted.

→ Use of examples very prematurely in sentences 2 and 3.
→ The fourth sentence is where the candidate answers question 1. This could have been written first to demonstrate their clear understanding of what is being asked.

By "self-inflicted diseases", the author may mean diseases such as CHD and liver cancer – diseases that are related to our lifestyle. By smoking and drinking excessive alcohol, people develop CHD and liver cancer. Obesity may also be considered because the obese person may have been eating large amounts of foods with a high cholesterol, fat and salt intake. On the other hand, people who are anorexic also damage their bodies by not eating enough. STIs may be considered as "self-inflicting", as well as attempted suicide, although suicide is physiological too.

→ CHD = "coronary heart disease". Avoid unnecessary abbreviations, write your answer for a general audience.
→ Some examples are good, others are used with caveats. To avoid this, one could talk in general terms first, and then select the most appropriate examples to illustrate ones point most effectively. This could be done in the planning stage.

Doctors treat people who have been in fights or in war, so why should they not treat people who have damaged their bodies by themselves? Regarding obesity, some obese people may not even eat that much, or attempt regular exercising. If doctors won't treat them why should they treat people who don't care about their health but still have a "non-inflicted" disease? Doctors are supposed to be caring – they should look out for the patient's wellbeing as well as treating them because psychological factors do have an influence. If the situation involves the risk of the patient dying, it is the doctor's responsibility to try and keep the patient alive, no matter what.

➔ The candidate has used rhetorical questions to attempt to make an argument with the use of examples. It would be more effective to leave the specific examples aside for a moment and to consider the underlying reasons used to support the conclusion.

- The example of obesity raises some issues which are heading towards some general points: the fact that it is difficult to call a disease self-inflicted because many people with that condition may suffer from it for no reason of their own doing (e.g. genetic).
- The candidate also uses a rhetorical question in getting to the point that if there are self-inflicted diseases there must be non-self-inflicted diseases and this is difficult to define.
- There are then some other points, again used with examples which attempt to argue from the stance that doctors have a duty to help people, no matter what caused their suffering.

Marker's Overall Comments

Generally this is satisfactory. The candidate has identified all three parts of the question and attempted to answer them in clearly designated paragraphs. There are some parts which could be better organised, which can be remedied by making a plan before answering. The answer to question 2 could be re-worked to be made much more effective. The answer to question 3 could also be re-worked to make a stronger argument; though many good thoughts are clearly present they could be developed. The overarching problem is the premature use of examples – the underlying points should be made and then backed-up by examples.

Score (1st Marker) = 6; (2nd Marker) = 9; Overall Score = 7.5

SAMPLE STUDENT ESSAY 2

I believe the statement is trying to convey that those diseases brought upon a patient by themselves should be perhaps given less priority as these diseases may have been warned against and advice by doctors and healthcare professionals may have been given. Therefore, if the warnings had not been taken into consideration, it is the patient's duty to look out for his own health and safety. It is simply ignorant to assume that sole reliance on the doctor is acceptable.

➔ This is a very good answer to question 1. Developed yet concise.

Some diseases which come under this heading would perhaps be obesity, even though it is not commonly thought of as a disease. Obesity is usually caused by one's own sedentary lifestyle such as lack of exercise, poor diet and possibly mental issues such as depression. Another example is smoking which causes many respiratory problems such as lung cancer, bronchitis and many other diseases. Alcohol and drug abuse are self-inflicted and cause damage to the liver, brain and potentially many other organs.

→ The candidate uses specific examples immediately without being general first.

However, these so-called "self-inflicted" diseases such as obesity are not always self-inflicted. Genetic and hereditary factors also play a part for some. Also, if someone is mentally depressed or in an unstable state of mind; they may seek comfort in cigarettes or alcohol. Therefore, this is not directly self-inflicted, so is denying proper treatment fair for this subgroup? It is the job of a doctor to preserve and look after the health of their nation, so no matter how a disease is caused, fair and unbiased treatment should always be provided. Therefore it is not fair for doctors to choose who receives treatment as was the case of a woman in need of a hip replacement, who was unfairly turned away until she lost enough weight. In conclusion, I believe that treatment should be given to all, but if it is the necessary to choose who receives immediate treatment, it would be the patient with the non-self-inflicted disease.

→ The candidate does make the argument here using obesity as an example. This could be better expressed in more general terms first.
→ The conclusion is not necessary. It also weakens the strength of the candidate's arguments since she backtracks to agree with the proposition she is supposed to be arguing against.

Marker's Overall Comments

The candidate has answered all three parts clearly and effectively. The answer to question 2 is the weakest. The rest is effective.

Score (1st Marker) = 9; (2nd Marker) = 12; Overall Score = 10.5

SAMPLE STUDENT ESSAY 3

The message that the statement conveys is that NHS doctors should not be permitted to treat people who have abused their health, and therefore those who are suffering with "self-inflicted" diseases are to be treated by other organisations. The author could also be suggesting this is because such patients are a waste of time and NHS money, which could be spent on patients who have other diseases and needs.

→ This is a very good answer to question 1.
→ It is also reflective and considers other implied meanings.

"Self-inflicted diseases" suggests that a patient's lifestyle has put them at risk of abusing their health. The author is inferring that this perhaps is deliberate or at least the patient is aware of the consequences, but they know the NHS will treat everyone, no matter what the circumstances. Some of these diseases could include smoking, obesity and conditions related to taking illegal substances.

→ This is a very good answer to question 2.
→ Although "smoking" is not a disease, we can give this candidate the benefit of the doubt because they obviously have a firm grasp of what they are talking about.

The treatment of self-inflicted diseases should be the responsibility of doctors in the NHS because a doctor should not be preoccupied with judging how their patient got the disease, but to treat it professionally. Segregating if diseases have been self-inflicted or not would first of all be difficult to define. It is not the doctor's job to interrogate the patient to discover if they prove it effectively either way. In addition the definition of "self-inflicted" could be applied to diseases arguably, and therefore the NHS would have less patients to treat, and more sick people left untreated.

Overall, it is a patient's prerogative to treat their bodies however they like, and lead a healthy, or unhealthy lifestyle. The NHS should not discriminate between patients this way because they provide a service and it is every patient's right to receive that service.

→ The answer to question 3 is very good. The opening statement (which is the argument's conclusion) cannot lead us anywhere else but to reasons supporting it. The complete absence of examples actually makes this answer stand out since very rarely can a candidate make such a

forceful argument without having to rely on (usually poor) examples. This demonstrates how examples are not essential to making an
argument, and leaves this candidate more time to make several strong
points to support the answer.

Marker's Overall Comments

A well-balanced, thoughtful and intelligent answer. Some examples in
answering question 3 may have made the answer even better, but it is better
to have no examples than to have poor or irrelevant examples. In any case
this does not detract from the overall high quality.

Score = 12

SAMPLE STUDENT ESSAY 4

> This statement is arguing that the treatment of certain diseases –
> termed "self-inflicted" – should not be provided by NHS doctors. The
> implication is that people are responsible to some extent for their
> own health and the consequences of their irresponsibility is a ration-
> ing of access to services (i.e. being seen/treated by an NHS doctor).

→ Very good answer. Concise yet complete.

> "Self-inflicted" probably refers to diseases caused by unwise life-
> style choices which are damaging to health and which are linked to
> disease which the person themselves have caused. I imagine those
> diseases linked to tobacco and alcohol would be included – e.g. cancer,
> heart and lung disease as well as fast foods and diet choices causing
> obesity.

→ Another excellently concise yet complete answer.

> One argument against this is as follows. Doctors are responsible for
> treating patients as part of the NHS. These patients pay taxes in
> order to receive healthcare. There is no rule stopping people from
> behaving in certain ways, even if damaging to health in a free society.
> Therefore NHS doctors should treat them regardless.
>   In addition, the premise has several flaws. It relies on the fact
> that the self-inflicted diseases are caused by "bad" behaviour and
> this link between may not be conclusive. If a particular disease has
> many causal factors, some of which are natural others are behav-
> ioural, distinguishing the actual cause would be impossible.

"Self-inflicted" also implies blame on the individual but disease may be caused through no fault of their own – e.g. by nature (genes) or the environment. Lack of knowledge that one particular behaviour caused disease would make it difficult to lay blame and label it "self-inflicted". Lack of knowledge may be due to poor education, poor memory (elderly or demented patients), mental illness or ignorance (i.e. an unknown risk which is subsequently found to be hazardous to health).

Also it could be argued to the extreme, that practically every lifestyle choice is hazardous to health. Therefore almost every possible health complaint could be deemed to be self-inflicted and no-one would qualify for NHS treatment as a result. Even accidents, which by definition cannot be self-inflicted, would count as self-inflicted – e.g. an injury from a car crash is self-inflicted because the lifestyle choice was to drive the car in the first place. A skiing injury is self-inflicted and so on.

→ Excellent! A very good way of beginning the answer to question 3 prepares us for the argument.
→ The answer is very good, contains many sound arguments and these are developed.
→ The candidate allocated their time and space wisely, leaving the most room to make polished arguments to question 3.

Marker's Overall Comments
This candidate has made an excellent attempt at an answer.

1 Well structured – in paragraphs
2 Concise and effective use of language
3 Answered all parts of the question very well – making clear points
4 Used examples adequately

Score = 15

SAMPLE STUDENT ESSAY 5

Essentially this statement means that those who have fallen ill as a result of their own lifestyle choices while fully knowing the consequences of these choices should not be the responsibility of doctors or the NHS.

In the statement this type of patient is said to have a "self-inflicted" disease. This can be summarised as a disease that the patient is either partially or fully responsible for falling victim to.

However, many would argue against the idea of responsibility being placed squarely on the shoulders of the patient. This as it is far too general and does not specify enough. It would therefore be almost impossible for a doctor to be the judge of who is worthy of treatment and who is not. On top of this there is no clear black and white regarding the concept of "self-inflicted diseases" and in certain scenarios would be very hard to judge whether a disease was self-inflicted or not. One could even argue that to an extent all diseases are self-inflicted.

Above all else it is the job of the NHS and doctors to help the ill regardless of the manner in which they fell ill.

Marker's Overall Comments

This candidate has clearly answered all three parts. It is very concise but the candidate has obviously a clear understanding of the issues. Although well argued, it could be more developed. This shows that it is not necessary to write a tome to have a decent answer.

Score = 9

SAMPLE STUDENT ESSAY 6

The statement is highly controversial and highlights an ethical problem within the NHS. It can relate to both injury caused by self-harm or to disease caused by ignorance or by will and states that the NHS doctors should not be responsible for treatment of this mainly due to the argument that patients should bear responsibility for their actions.

However there are multiple arguments to dispute this, one of note is that the NHS should treat all people indiscriminately. It is not fair to refuse people treatment on the grounds the injury was self-inflicted, either due to lack of education or mental problems as this will neglect a group of society. There have been many protests against discrimination showing public support of this argument; this public funds the NHS. Patients who self-inflict an illness are often not to blame. Many reasons are out of the patients control such as the education they had or the money they earn.

It then is not fair to refuse treatment to them when they were not at fault. A final point is that the NHS was set up to provide treatment to those who do not have the money for private treatment. To refuse patients, who very well may not have the money for treatment, on any grounds goes against the reason for the NHS and so the treatments of these patients should be the responsibility of doctors in the NHS.

Marker's Overall Comments

It is not clear that the candidate has answered questions 1 and 2. Although they have been combined in the first paragraph, it would be better to distinctly separate these. The rest of the argument is relatively well done, although not very well expressed.

Score = 6

SAMPLE STUDENT ESSAY 7

This statement is saying that self-inflicted diseases should not be the responsibility of doctors in the NHS but it should be the responsibility of the person who has inflicted pain onto themselves. When the author says "self-inflicted diseases", I think ~~he~~ they meant things like ~~a drugs overdose where it is the choice of the person to take it and self inflict harm~~ smoking where the effects of this are clearly displayed on packaging and other media like ~~emphysema and bronchitis~~ e.g. ~~newspapers~~ on the news. People have had an increasing awareness of diseases like emphysema and bronchitis since the introduction of media to help raise public awareness but as some people choose to waste their money buying cigarettes, they are self-inflicting disease among themselves. Also obesity and its associated diseases, e.g. CHD, where an introduction to a change in healthier eating ~~is trying~~, in schools especially, by Jamie Oliver, is self-inflicted as people may choose to ignore advice. However, I think that the doctor role is to help and cure patients with the aim of improving their quality of life and they should not judge whether the patient has self-inflicted or not. The NHS is available to anyone seeking medical attention and has done so for about 55 years. It is known that there are increasing STDs being spread and it could be seen that these are self-inflicted but it is still the duty of the doctor to treat the patient to improve their life and maybe prevent others from also contracting the disease. Could it be argued that genetic diseases like sickle cell anaemia are self-inflicted and don't deserve treatment ~~as the~~ if the parents knew their child might contract the disease? ~~Most d~~ Some diseases could be argued are self-inflicted which will be perceived differently by everyone and so doctors should treat self-inflicted diseases, as they treat other diseases.

Marker's Overall Comments

Clearly not planned in advance. The candidate has used language very ineffectively and has disadvantaged himself by wasting space with crossings-out. Also their focus on irrelevant examples is unnecessary. Although they have answered all parts of the question, it is disorganised and at a fairly simplistic level.

Score = 6

Now take a look at the following three questions, and before reading the sample (unedited) student answers of varying standard, try answering them for yourself under timed exam conditions. Then score the sample answers using the scoring system outlined above and compare these to your answer and score your own attempt.

Example Question 2

Under no circumstances should the primary principle guiding a doctor's practice, of "primum non nocere" ("first, do no harm"), be ignored.

Write a unified essay in which you address the following:

1 Explain what you think this statement means.
2 Why should this be the fundamental principle to which doctors adhere?
3 Advance an argument against the statement above, i.e. "under certain circumstances the primary principle guiding a doctor's practice, of *'primum non nocere'* ('first, do no harm') may be ignored."

  – *Before reading further attempt the question for yourself, under exam conditions.*

SAMPLE STUDENT ESSAY 1

The statement given clearly supports the most important set of principles a doctor must abide by given in the Hippocratic Oath. As a doctor's job is to care for the patient and treat them with respect and dignity, the statement is emphasising the need for a doctor to judge a patient's symptoms, diagnose and treat without causing any harm. There is no need to cut a patients skin to remove a lump for laboratory analysis if clearly it is a benign cyst. The doctor should never "do harm" as a first resort but use their skills and experience of anatomy and physiology to know the body and possible reasons for an illness.

Doctors should adhere to this principle as teachers, social workers and all other members of authority and responsibility must take, in situations of possible abuse, or times when the doctor is unsure of what a symptom may be caused by. Professional advice, from colleagues or other sources should always be the first method – reducing the risk of infection, limiting/conserving funds of the NHS and also reducing the risk of legal battles if patients were wrongly cut.

Situations that may contradict the principle and therefore result in "first, do no harm" being ignored, may be rare but crucial to a patient's health. A doctor in A+E or one called to an emergency which could lead to imminent fatalities, should use their intuition and consult any other doctors/nurses/paramedics but cut or insert needles or remove substances if need be at the time. Often instincts combined with a rush of adrenaline (as humans need for survival) will override a principle which in practice is not practical in a critical situation. A risk of infection in order to save or elongate someone's life by cutting at a malignant melanoma instantly may seem controversial but fulfils the main role of a doctor – to put the health and lives of their patients first.

YOUR COMMENTS:

YOUR SCORE:

Example Question 3

Doctors can do as much harm by telling the truth to their patients as they can by lying. Therefore there are circumstances which exist when lying to one's patients is acceptable.

Write a unified essay in which you address the following:

1 Explain what you think this statement means.
2 What circumstances do you think the author had in mind?
3 Advance an argument against the statement above, i.e. "there are not circumstances which exist when lying to one's patients is acceptable"

   –Before reading further attempt the question for yourself, under exam conditions.

SAMPLE STUDENT ESSAY 1

Doctors are seen as trusted members of society, who would usually have the ability to see problems with an individual's health thus a reputation to uphold credibility. However, it is sometimes necessary for a doctor to lie to their patients to protect their wellbeing.

An example of this would be in the case of a young child diagnosed with a terminal disease. Or, an individual that may harm themselves as a result of finding out that they may die or be ill. Harm may be characterised as taking their own life or even taking others' lives in the desperation of being saved. In the case of the child it is better to leave the child in happiness over its last few days. If one weren't to lie to the child it may in fact suffer from severe depression causing unnecessary trauma to the entire family. If the problem existed on a larger scale, i.e. if the disease was life threatening and highly contagious doctors should quarantine the infected individual and lie to the media to prevent widespread panic and possibly damaging effects to the health service and economy.

On the contrary referring back to the earlier point of a doctor's credibility, the patient expects the doctor to be honest, especially with the widespread knowledge regarding the Hippocratic Oath. If the patient later found out that the doctor had lied that patient may hold a misconception of all doctors and refuse consultations and treatment in future. However, the benefits of lying in certain circumstances outweigh the problems. Therefore lying in certain circumstances is acceptable.

YOUR COMMENTS:

YOUR SCORE:

EXAMPLE QUESTION 4

Scientific research should only be carried out if it is likely to produce an increase in knowledge directly or indirectly relevant to the benefit of humankind.

Write a unified essay in which you address the following:

1 Explain what you think this statement means.
2 What justification can be used to support this view?
3 Advance an argument against the statement above, i.e. "Research should not only be carried out if it is likely to produce an increase in knowledge directly or indirectly relevant to the benefit of humankind."

   –Before reading further attempt the question for yourself, under exam conditions.

SAMPLE STUDENT ESSAY 1

The statement implies that scientific research should only be under-taken if the research is likely to create knowledge which is relevant to the benefit of mankind. The benefit of mankind can be seen as an increase in people's quality of life or length of life. The scientific research into the movements of distant galaxies, for example, would arguably not produce such beneficial knowledge.

The argument is justifiable. Scientific development in areas which are detrimental to mankind can be seen as unethical because they may reduce people's quality and length of life, and increase suffering. Scientific research which is into fields which are neither beneficial to mankind nor harmful can also be seen as unethical. Scientific research is expensive and requires a lot of specialist manpower, and scientists are rare. As well as wasting resources, fields of research irrelevant to the benefit of mankind could pull these resources from potentially relevant areas, thus reducing the amount of research into useful fields.

However, the counterargument can be justified. Research into areas which are harmful can produce beneficial results. An example is the creation of radar, which was originally for military use, but is now employed in many civilian ways, such as landing planes safely.

YOUR COMMENTS:

YOUR SCORE:

SAMPLE STUDENT ESSAY 2

This statement makes a distinction between three types of knowledge: knowledge which is directly/indirectly relevant to benefit mankind which I call "useful"; other knowledge is either "useless" but still neutral, or actually positively harmful which I term "bad."

The statement supports research only for the first type of knowledge acquisition. The implications are that the others are not worth pursuing.

Possible justifications basically rely on the fact that there is a shortage of resources – time, money, expertise and a desire towards self-preservation. Thus:

1 Research is expensive and someone has to fund it. Research into weapons or war machines for example, and other harmful things ("bad" research) should not be funded as they are a waste of the limited resource money.
2 Researchers are in short supply so why waste time on researching "useless" or "bad" subjects – assuming the aim is to benefit humankind and advance.
3 We don't want harm to come to us via knowledge acquisition – self-preservation.
4 There is also a paternalistic justification, i.e. someone has to decide what constitutes a direct or indirect benefit to humankind, and that may be seen as a caring force (be it government, a scientific committee, or whoever looking out for our interests).

To counter these assertions, the distinction made in the statement about knowledge is a false one. All research is neutral until humans add particular value to it. For example, the desire for self-preservation should not stop research since it is the use of results of research and not research itself which could cause the harm. Humans are rational animals able to make decisions based on the research findings. The fact that there is potential for research to be carried out into "useless" or "bad" avenues shouldn't stop the quest for knowledge before it is begun because (1) knowledge pursuit as an intellectual activity is uniquely human and should be encouraged and stimulated, (2) so-called "useless" knowledge may one day be useful, so excluding it from the research scope now is short sighted and unintelligent (possibly harmful), (3) knowledge pursuit is enjoyable for those who do it, and in a free society the democratic system should allow them to research what they like.

YOUR COMMENTS:

YOUR SCORE:

Part D: Summary

Common mistakes (in no particular order)

The following list has been created after marking hundreds of student's essays (like the ones shown in this chapter) and noting the mistakes which are most consistently made.

By pointing these out to you we hope to help you avoid making them yourselves.

1 Lack of planning

You may think that you have points to make; in the heat of the moment you may think that you have more to say than you actually do; you may even have several half-thoughts (which do not amount to much when you write them down). You then start writing your final answer immediately, so that these half-thoughts do not leave you, without making a plan of the whole question from start to finish first. The end result is a disorganised disaster. Don't break the cardinal rule: plan!

2 Arguments

Remember that an *argument* is *reasons* supporting a *conclusion* (from Critical Thinking). As you have seen in the example questions in this chapter, you will usually be given one viewpoint and you will have to make an argument against a proposed statement or viewpoint.

Since this can be difficult to construct under time pressure this is frequently the least well answered part of the question. You therefore must spend time whilst making a plan concentrating on how to make the argument for that particular question. By considering all the questions you can see which argument you can make most convincingly. If you can answer the argument part of the question, the other parts are usually more straightforward and you will score well.

3   Examples

Introducing examples is best avoided until after you have finished planning your answer. Examples are not arguments but frequently examples are used by students mistakenly as arguments. Usually the same example is used by every candidate; this is not a great problem but being original will help your answer to stand out. Because, in the heat of the moment, the examples given can be bizarre, over-specific (and hence usually long-winded), irrelevant or limited to your own experience they are therefore best avoided. Examples are easy to think of so don't concentrate on them until you have written a sound piece which can then be improved by carefully selected illustrative examples.

4   Poor structure

You answer the question but in a disjointed or disorganised way. The answer is not easy to read and does not flow logically from one part to the next. This shows a lack of organised thought. This could be solved by making a plan with clear points which are correctly ordered before writing.

5   Incomplete

You answer the question in part but there are essential parts missing. This could be solved by making a plan with clear points indicating answers to all parts of question before writing. Incomplete answers will not score highly.

6   Unbalanced

You answer the question fully but there is too much written in response to one or more parts of the question *at the expense of another part(s)*. You want to spend most of the time and space writing the argument. This is the most difficult part, so a good answer here will shine through. If the question is divided into a "What" part (e.g. "What do you think this statement means?") then this should be a short couple of sentences. There is no need to start elaborating on a relatively minor or straightforward part of the question.

7   Digression (wandering off point)

You include irrelevant details which have no bearing on the question and are a waste of space. This shows a lack of organised thinking. At the extreme this can be answering a different question. Not a good move (but surprisingly, not that rare!) This could be solved by making a plan before writing.

8   Waffle (not being concise)

Usually due to a paucity of relevant points to make. This may be because the wrong question was chosen. This could be solved by making a plan before answering the question, where a lack of points to make would have been apparent.

9   Repeating the same point in a different way

You may not realise you have done this. If you plan your answer and number each distinct and specific point you are going to make, it won't happen.

10   Writing too much

If you write more than the allotted space it will not get marked. You may therefore lose credit if vital parts of your answer are on the unmarked overrun pages.

Quick test

1 What does the Writing Task test?
2 To what other part of the BMAT is the Writing Task similar, and how?
3 What schema should you use when approaching the Writing Task?
4 What is the single most important thing to do when answering the Writing Task question?
5 *True or false*: Bullet points and subheadings can be very useful in answering the writing task.

CHAPTER 5

Abstract reasoning for the UKCAT

Part A: First glance

In this part of the test you are presented with two sets of shapes, labelled Set A and Set B, to look at and consider. In each Set there are six different panels. Each panel in Set A is there because it follows a specific rule. Similarly, each panel in Set B is there because it follows a *different* rule. You have to work out what these rules are by observation and deduction. In other words, there is something in common with all the shapes in Set A. And there is a *different* common feature for all the shapes in Set B.

You are given test shapes which you have place into either Set A or Set B using the rules you have decided operate. You do this by asking yourself, "Does the test shape follow the rule for Set A? Or Set B? Or Neither?" If the test shapes cannot be placed into Set A or Set B, you choose "Neither" as the answer.

In what circumstance is "neither" the correct answer?

In just two general circumstances:

1 The test shape follows the rule for Set A *and* it also follows the rule for Set B. In this case you cannot reliably place it in either Set, so the safest (and correct) option is neither.
2 The test shape does not follow the rule for Set A *or* the rule for Set B. So it follows a different rule which does not belong in either Set. So "neither" is the appropriate response.

Part B: The approach

For example: In the question below consider the panels in Set A. *Remember*: Each panel in Set A is there because it follows a specific rule. Use careful observation and thought to decide what that rule is. By looking at all the panels in Set A, you can see that each panel contains white circles. The rule for Set A seems to be that each panel must be composed of white circles.

Now look at the panels in Set B. Again remember: each panel in Set B is there because it follows a specific rule (which is *different* to the rule for Set A). By observation and thought you can see that each panel contains black circles. The rule for Set B seems to be that each panel must be composed of black circles.

Now, happy with the rules for Set A and set B in your mind, look at each test shape in turn and ask yourself, "Does the test shape follow the rule for Set A? Or Set B? Or Both? Or Neither?"

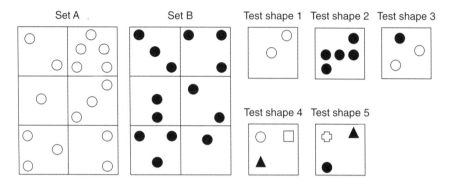

This is a very simple example. It relied only on the *colour* of the objects being different, and this simple fact determined the rule. There can be other factors around which rules can be constructed which we will consider later.

	Set A	Set B	
General rule	Colour of circles	Colour of circles	
Specific rule	All the circles are white	All the circles are black	
Option	**Comment**		**Answer**
Test shape 1	All the circles are white. So it follows the rule for Set A.		*Set A*
Test shape 2	All the circles are black. So it follows the rule for Set B.		*Set B*
Test shape 3	This contains white circles and black circles. So it does not follow either the rule for Set A or the rule for Set B. So the answer is "neither".		*Neither*
Test shape 4	This contains other shapes. So it does not follow either the rule for Set A or the rule for Set B. So the answer is "neither".		*Neither*
Test shape 5	This contains other shapes. So it does not follow either the rule for Set A or the rule for Set B. So the answer is "neither".		*Neither*

Quick test

Put yourself in the shoes of a question setter for a moment. If you were making these questions, think about how the shapes can be organised. What general rules might there be? How about more specific rules? How can we arrange shapes according to simple rules? What about more complex rules?

Spend some time thinking about ways in which you might like to organise shapes, and list them in the table below:

1	6
2	7
3	8
4	9
5	10

What did you come up with?

General ways like the number, shape, colour, rotation of shapes, the number of sides a shape has, its position in the panel. Also for each of these general rules, we can think about more specific rules.

Number: odd numbers of shapes, even number of shapes, the same number of shapes per panel etc.

Shape: the same shapes used in each panel, or unique shapes used each time, etc.

Colour/pattern: each shape the same colour or each box contains 50% black and 50% white shapes, unique patterning for each shape, etc.

And many more . . .

It can be easy to spot a simple rule, but you must look more closely and think if there are other more subtle rules.

Part C: Practice

Look at the two worked examples below. Then try to do the other questions for yourself (answers are given at the end of this chapter).

Item 1

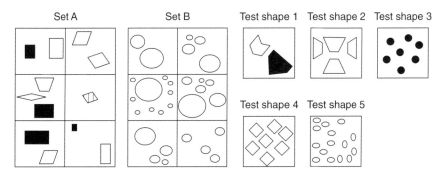

	Set A	Set B	
General rule	Number of sides	Number of white circles	
Specific rule	All the shapes have four sides	An even number of circles	
Option	**Comment**		**Answer**
Test shape 1	The shapes do not follow either rule.		*Neither*
Test shape 2	All the shapes have four sides		*Set A*
Test shape 3	There are black circles and an odd number (7).		*Neither*
Test shape 4	The shapes are four sided.		*Set A*
Test shape 5	There are white circles but an odd number (15).		*Neither*

If you are finding it difficult to come up with the rule, start by looking at the most basic panel in the Set. For example, in Item 1 above, Set A only has a single shape in the middle right hand panel.

Remember, in order for a panel to be included in a Set, it must follow a clear rule.

So any rule which applies to Set A has to apply to the most basic panel as well as the more complex ones. This will act as a starting point in deciding the rules for any Set.

In this case there is a single four-sided shape, positioned just left of centre, with some diagonal shading. What aspect of these facts links it to the rule? Once you have an idea, start to test this by looking at other panels in Set A and see if there are common features. In this way you can build up a rule. Test it with each panel; if it does not fit any of the panels then it is not the rule: and you must think again.

The rule for Set A must be different for Set B. If you see common features between both sets, then that cannot be the rule.

Item 2

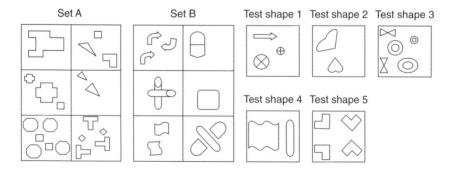

	Set A	Set B	
General rule 1	Type of shapes	Type of shapes	
Specific rule 1	All the shapes have straight lines	All the shapes are made up of both straight *and* curved parts	
Option	**Comment**		**Answer**
Test shape 1	There are two shapes with curved lines and straight lines (Set B) but one shape with straight lines only (Set A). Therefore we cannot assign it to either Set with confidence.		*Neither*
Test shape 2	There are two shapes which each have straight and curved lines.		*Set B*
Test shape 3	There are shapes composed of curves alone and shapes composed of lines alone. These are feature of both Sets.		*Neither*
Test shape 4	There are curves and straight lines in each shape.		*Set B*
Test shape 5	The shapes are composed of lines only.		*Set A*

Item 3

Set A	Set B	Test shape 1	Test shape 2	Test shape 3

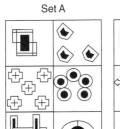 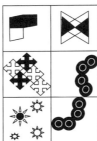 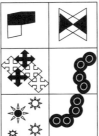 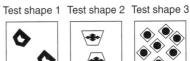 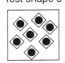 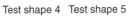

Test shape 4   Test shape 5

	Set A	Set B	
General rule			
Specific rule			
Option	**Comment**		**Answer**
Test shape 1			
Test shape 2			
Test shape 3			
Test shape 4			
Test shape 5			

Item 4

Set A   Set B   Test shape 1 Test shape 2 Test shape 3

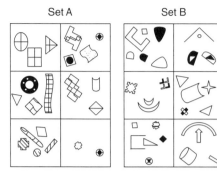
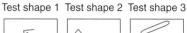
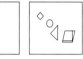

Test shape 4 Test shape 5

	Set A	Set B	
General rule			
Specific rule			
Option	Comment		Answer
Test shape 1			
Test shape 2			
Test shape 3			
Test shape 4			
Test shape 5			

Item 5

Set A   Set B   Test shape 1 Test shape 2 Test shape 3

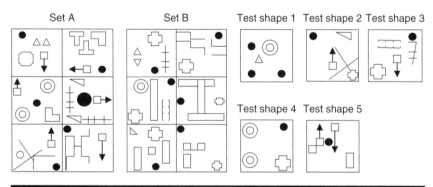

	Set A	Set B	
General rule			
Specific rule			
Option	Comment		Answer
Test shape 1			
Test shape 2			
Test shape 3			
Test shape 4			
Test shape 5			

Item 6

Set A	Set B	Test shape 1	Test shape 2	Test shape 3

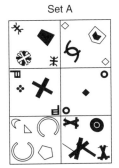 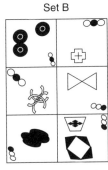 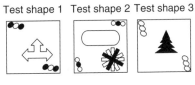

Test shape 4	Test shape 5

	Set A	Set B	
General rule			
Specific rule			
Option	**Comment**		**Answer**
Test shape 1			
Test shape 2			
Test shape 3			
Test shape 4			
Test shape 5			

Item 7

Set A	Set B	Test shape 1	Test shape 2	Test shape 3

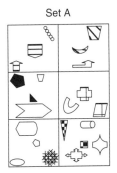 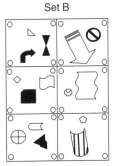 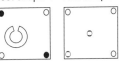

Test shape 4	Test shape 5

	Set A	Set B	
General rule			
Specific rule			
Option	**Comment**		**Answer**
Test shape 1			
Test shape 2			
Test shape 3			
Test shape 4			
Test shape 5			

Item 8

	Set A	Set B
	Set A	Set B
	Set A			Test shape 1	Test shape 2	Test shape 3

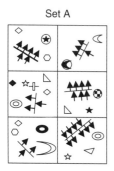 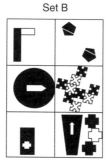 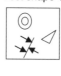 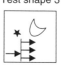

Test shape 4   Test shape 5

	Set A		**Set B**	
General rule				
Specific rule				
Option	**Comment**			**Answer**
Test shape 1				
Test shape 2				
Test shape 3				
Test shape 4				
Test shape 5				

Item 9

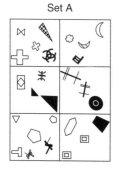 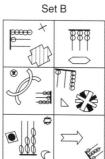 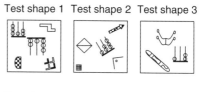

Test shape 4   Test shape 5

	Set A		**Set B**	
General rule				
Specific rule				
Option	**Comment**			**Answer**
Test shape 1				
Test shape 2				
Test shape 3				
Test shape 4				
Test shape 5				

Item 10

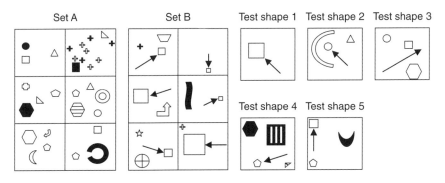

	Set A		Set B	
General rule				
Specific rule				
Option	**Comment**			**Answer**
Test shape 1				
Test shape 2				
Test shape 3				
Test shape 4				
Test shape 5				

It is important not just to spot the rules but to learn to *articulate* them. This will help prevent you being caught out when the rules are very subtle.

Part D: Answers

Item 3	Set A	Set B
General rule 1	Colour of shapes	Colour of shapes
Specific rule 1	All the shapes have an inner black component with an outer white surround.	All the shapes have a black-and-white component (in any combination).
General rule 2	Number of shapes.	There is no 2nd rule for Set B.
Specific rule 2	There is an odd number of shapes in each box.	There is no 2nd rule for Set B.
Option	**Comment**	**Answer**
Test shape 1	The shapes have a black-and-white component (Set B). The specific pattern does not follow the rule for Set A.	*Set B*

Option	Comment	Answer
Test shape 2	Although there is a black inner component and a white outer component to the shapes (Set A rule 1) there are two shapes (Set A rule 2 = must contain an odd number of shapes). It does have a black-and-white component (Set B).	*Set B*
Test shape 3	There is a black inner component and a white outer component (Set A). Also there are 7 shapes (rule 2) (Set A).	*Set A*
Test shape 4	There is a single black object. There are no white objects.	*Neither*
Test shape 5	*Colour*: only white. Therefore neither rule.	*Neither*

Item 4	Set A		Set B
General rule	Shapes		Shapes
Specific rule	Each shape in the panel is unique.		One example of a large shape "eating" a smaller shape.

Option	Comment	Answer
Test shape 1	There are two examples of shapes "eating" smaller ones.	*Neither*
Test shape 2	All the shapes are unique.	*Set A*
Test shape 3	There is a shape "eating" a smaller one (Set B). But all the shapes are unique (Set A). Both rules apply.	*Neither*
Test shape 4	There is a shape trying to "eat" another shape but it is too big – and therefore does *not* follow the rule for Set B. The shapes *are* unique (Set A).	*Set A*
Test shape 5	There is a shape eating two smaller ones.	*Neither*

Item 5	Set A		Set B
General rule 1	Shape		Shape
Specific rule 1	Solid circle shape and a square-with-arrow shape.		White cross and filled circle.
General rule 2	Relative position		Relative position
Specific rule 2	The position of the circle relative to the square determines the direction of the arrow: it always points away from the circle: e.g. when the circle is above the square the arrow is *down*, when the circle is below, the arrow is *up*, when they are horizontally aligned the arrow points away from the circle horizontally.		The filled circle and the white cross are always oppositely positioned with respect to one another.

Option	Comment	Answer
Test shape 1	The panel contains three solid circles but no square-with-arrow shapes (Set A) or white crosses (Set B).	*Neither*

Option	Comment	Answer
Test shape 2	The filled circle and the white cross are positioned in opposite corners (Set B). Although the square-with-arrow shape is present it does not follow the rule for Set A so its presence can be said to be incidental.	*Set B*
Test shape 3	The filled circle and the white cross are positioned in opposite corners (Set B). And the square-with-arrow shape follows the rule for Set A. These are feature of both Sets.	*Neither*
Test shape 4	The filled circle and the white cross are positioned opposite one another.	*Set B*
Test shape 5	The square-with-arrow shape and the filled circle are present but do not follow the rule for Set A.	*Neither*

Item 6	Set A	Set B
General rule 1	Shape	Shape
Specific rule 1	Identical shapes appear in opposite corners.	The three-circles-shape is positioned in one corner only.
General rule 2	There is no 2nd rule for Set A.	Colour
Specific rule 2	There is no 2nd rule for Set A.	The three-circles-shape has two open and one filled colour pattern, (in any combination).

Option	Comment	Answer
Test shape 1	There is a three-circles-shape in opposite corners. This follows Set A's rule.	*Set A*
Test shape 2	The three-circles-shape (correctly represented (two open, one filled)) appear in both corners. This is not the rule for Set B, but a correctly applied rule for Set A since they are identical shapes.	*Set A*
Test shape 3	An exact shape represented in both corners = Set A.	*Set A*
Test shape 4	Follow Set B rule.	*Set B*
Test shape 5	Follows Set B rule.	*Set B*

Item 7	Set A	Set B
General rule 1	Position	Position
Specific rule 1	Central and corner shape.	Each corner has a circle
General rule 2	Colour	Colour
Specific rule 2	The shapes' patterns are identical.	The circle is white

Option	Comment	Answer
Test shape 1	The four corners are not white circles.	*Neither*
Test shape 2	The rule for Set A is followed.	*Set A*
Test shape 3	The rule for Set A is followed.	*Set A*
Test shape 4	Both rules are followed.	*Neither*
Test shape 5	Follows Set B rule.	*Set B*

Item 8	Set A	Set B	
General rule 1	Shape	Colour	
Specific rule 1	The arrow-and-line conformations are present in each panel.	Each panel has at least one black-and-white shape.	
General rule 2	Number	Relative proportions	
Specific rule 2	The number of arrows pointing towards the line are less than the number pointing away from the line.	Each black-and-white shape is comprised of more black than white shading.	
General rule 3	Orientation	There is no 3rd rule for Set B.	
Specific rule 3	The arrows point in the same direction in each individual conformation.	There is no 3rd rule for Set B.	
Option	**Comment**		**Answer**
Test shape 1	The arrows are not pointing in the correct directions to fulfil Set A's rule 3. Nor is there more black than white (Set B).		*Neither*
Test shape 2	The arrows do not fulfil Set A's rule. More black is present.		*Set B*
Test shape 3	The arrows follow the Set A rule.		*Set A*
Test shape 4	Set A's rule 2 is not followed. Set B's rule 2 is not followed.		*Neither*
Test shape 5	The rules for Set A and Set B are fulfilled.		*Neither*
Item 9	Set A	Set B	
General rule 1	Shape	Shape	
Specific rule 1	Two identical shapes used.	One "abacus" shape is present.	
General rule 2	Position	Number	
Specific rule 2	The central shape is also present in one of the corners.	The "abacus" has a total of six beads on it.	
Option	**Comment**		**Answer**
Test shape 1	The abacus shape is included, with six beads, but also repeated in the corner (i.e. both rules).		*Neither*
Test shape 2	The abacus with six beads follows the rule for Set B.		*Set B*
Test shape 3	The abacus shape is represented but does not have a total of six beads (not the rule for Set B). The rule for Set A is also not followed.		*Neither*
Test shape 4	The shape in the centre appears in the corner also.		*Set A*
Test shape 5	The abacus shape is seen but the beads do not equal six. Therefore this is not the rule for Set B. The central shape is repeated in the corner (Set A).		*Set A*

Item 10	Set A	Set B
General rule 1	Shapes	Shape
Specific rule 1	Several shapes are present with different numbers of sides.	Arrow pointing to a square.
General rule 2	Number	There is no 2nd rule for Set B.
Specific rule 2	At least some shapes have consecutive numbers of sides.	There is no 2nd rule for Set B.

Option	Comment	Answer
Test shape 1	The rule for Set B: an arrow pointing to a square.	*Set B*
Test shape 2	The arrow is pointing at a circle. There is not a four-sided shape present (i.e. consecutive number of sides with a triangle).	*Neither*
Test shape 3	There is an arrow present, but it is not pointing at the square. So it does not follow the rule for Set B. There are two regular shapes – a square and a hexagon. These have four and six sides, respectively, but they do not have a "consecutive number of sides". So this is not the rule for Set A either.	*Neither*
Test shape 4	The shapes – a triangle, square, pentagon and hexagon – all have a consecutive number of sides. This is the rule for Set A. The arrow present points at a pentagon, not a square (i.e. not the rule for Set B).	*Set A*
Test shape 5	There is an arrow present which points to a square (Set B). But also present in the box is a five-sided shape – i.e. there is a four- and five-sided shape present (Set A). Since there are components of both Set A and Set B we cannot assign the test shape to either Set with certainty.	*Neither*

Take care: Never forget that you have a third choice apart from Set A and Set B. Choice C (i.e. Neither Set A nor Set B, or both) is the correct answer if the rule for the Test Shape follows both rules at the same time or is completely new.

CHAPTER 6

Decision analysis for the UKCAT

Part A: First glance

The Decision Analysis part of the test can be broken down into two parts: analysis and decision making. In this part of the test, you are presented with a code list and are asked to decode or encode various items. The first problem to solve is to look at the code list and analyse it carefully. Following a logical and systematic analysis, you can eliminate wrong answers and narrow down the choices to two or three possibilities. Since there are sometimes more than one acceptable answer, you have to judge the best answer. You then make a decision about the best answer. Since all the questions are based on the same codes so you have extra time to spend on the code itself before answering the questions.

Part B: The approach

It is best to look at an example.

Example code:

General rules	Basic codes
P = opposite	305 = stop
Q = positive	306 = speak
R = total	307 = vehicle

Part I: Analysis

Step 1

Carefully read through the code list. It is likely that there are words that have more than one possible interpretation, or which at first glance have only one meaning, but with further thought (or even lateral thinking) further interpretations can be "squeezed" out.

For example the word "positive" may refer to size, number, attitude, mood, etc.

The word "total" may mean "everything", "all", "whole", "full", or we may squeeze out other meanings like "lots", "sum", "add", etc.

Obviously if we have an open mind (and a large vocabulary) we may be able to imagine translations which are very tenuous. But we should be aware of these and consider them, however unlikely – because they may be the best translation available. In these situations the answer options will act as prompts as to how much you can stretch a meaning.

Another example of when we may squeeze out a meaning:

"Word" – this could loosely mean speech or language, possibly a newspaper or book (written words) or TV or radio (spoken word) in the right context.

Quick test

Think of words which have more than one meaning and other words which you have to "squeeze" other meanings out of.

Step 2
Look at the question and for each code begin with a completely literal decoding.

Step 3
Pay careful attention to the position of the *commas* or other separators (such as *brackets*). These will tell you which parts of the code belong together.

Step 4
Look at the your translation, and consider possible meanings which have been created following the separators being factored into the translation.

Step 5
Compare this to the options. You should be able to eliminate several options. Wrong answers tend to have a predictable format and you should be on the look out for common ways the question-setters can try to fool you.

Part II: Decision making

Step 6
After the analysis, it is more than likely that you have spotted the wrong answer choices and the correct answer is clear. However, sometimes there may be more than one answer which appears to translate the code adequately. If this is the case, first double check that you have not mistranslated during the analysis. If your analysis is sound, then this is where you have to exercise judgement and choose the most sensible answer (i.e. make a decision!).

With the remaining options, consider which makes most sense – ask yourself, "if someone were to say one of these things to me, which would make most sense (or seem least odd)?"

Do remember though that one answer is clearly considered correct somewhere in the options.

Worked Example

What is the best interpretation of the following coded message: R, 307, P(305), QQ.

Part I: Analysis

Step 1

Look at the codes. Some potential problems may arise from words which can have several interpretations, such as the word "total", which may mean "all, everything, sum," etc.

Step 2

Literal decoding.

R	307	P	305	Q	Q
Total	Vehicle	Opposite	Stop	Positive	Positive

Step 3

Take care to pay attention to the separators, to improve the sense of the sentence.

R	307	P(305)	QQ
Total	Vehicle	Opposite (Stop)	Positive positive

Step 4

Re-evaluate in light of the steps 1 and 3.

Opposite(stop) = go; don't stop; not stop; non stop.

Positive positive = very positive; very much; lots; very big; very fast; very happy.

Step 5

Compare your translation to the options:

A All the vehicles on the road were going too fast
B The car was not stopping as fast as possible
C Every vehicle stopped very very slowly
D The whole vehicle was moving at an exceptional speed
E All the motorbikes went very fast

Option	General wrong-answer feature	Explanation
A	New word/concept	The word "road" has appeared. This is not in the code. *Even though it still makes sense it is not an accurate translation and so is incorrect.*
B	Ignored word/concept	The concept represented by "R" – "total" is not in this translation. *This is not the best answer because it is incomplete.*
C	Mistranslation	P(305) has been mistranslated as "stop" rather than "opposite stop". It seems that opposite has been wrongly applied to "QQ" – which has produced "very very slowly". The separators have not been correctly identified.
D	Not the best translation	A literal translation which makes sense, but does not sound fluent. This is where the decision making is applied.

Option E is an accurate translation ("motorbike" has been "squeezed" out of "vehicle") and sounds better than option D.

Part II: Decision making

Step 6

In this example, following the analysis, we are left with two possible answers to decide between.

Most people would agree that option E is the best answer out of the two choices.

Note, if there was a part of option E which was clearly mistranslated then option D would be correct, even if it sounds a little unnatural: a completely correct answer which sounds funny is still better than a fluent but incorrect answer!

Part way through the test the code list is expanded. The new codes are used in combination with the original codes to broaden the repertoire of questions that can be asked.

Expanded code list:

General rules	Basic codes
P = opposite	305 = stop
Q = positive	306 = speak
R = total	307 = vehicle
S = dress	308 = red
T = mood	309 = short
U = diet	310 = woman

Part of the decision making test is to start with a translation and asking you to choose from several codes the best code option to represent it. This is the same process as decoding, but done in reverse.

The most straightforward way to ensure an accurate translation is to consider all the possible options, and carefully translate by following the 6 steps as above. You will find that literally decoding the options is the only sure-fire way of not making a mistake.

Worked example: What would be the best way to encode the following message: The angry man wore red shorts.

A T, P(310), S, 308(309)
B 310, S, 308, 309
C S(308), P(310), 309, P(QT)
D QT, 306(QU), P(310), S
E PQ(T), P(310), S, 308(309)

By carefully following the steps for literal decoding, one can see that the options will, as before, have common mistake patterns. One important consideration is to look at the translation and consider the potential problems with words which may not be on the code list as a direct translation and how meanings may be "squeezed" into the possible answer.

Option	General wrong-answer feature	Explanation
A	Missing concept	The idea of "mood" is represented by "T" but there is no modifier to suggest anger.
B	Mistranslation	310 is wrongly translated as "woman" – but we need "man".
C	Wrong separators	S(308) has been put together which is not the best coded translation.
D	New concept	The word "treat" represented by "306" has been introduced, which is not required.

Option E is an accurate translation and most appropriate.

Quick test

Option D in the worked example above has more than one wrong-answer feature. There is the introduction of a new concept, but what else is wrong?

Another style of question asks if there are other codes which would be useful to add to the code list in order to allow the accurate translation of a given phrase. The addition of more than one word may be required. Approaching such a question, you should ask whether the words in the question can be encoded from the existing codes; if not, this is a possible option for the answer.

Example: Which of the following would be the most useful and the second most useful additions to the codes in order to convey the message accurately?

Message: None of us could sleep for long because everyone was woken by the loud shouting.

A Able
B Everyone
C Shout
D Sleep
E Wake

In the question above, consider the words in the options **A** to **E**, and see if these can be translated using the existing codes.

Option	Comment
A Able	No clear way of obtaining by using existing codes: possible answer
B Everyone	Could be obtained by "total" (R)
C Shout	Could be squeezed out of "speak" (306) and modified with "positive" (Q) (i.e. speak louder – shout)
D Sleep	No way of encoding – possible answer
E Wake	No way of encoding – possible answer

The analysis has lead to three possible answers. However, "sleep" and "wake" are opposites, so one could be chosen and the other obtained from applying "P" – "opposite". And the other option "able" can be chosen. So the answer here would be A and D or E.

Although there are other words which may not be represented by the codes (like the small/linking words (e.g. us, for, because)), the options only include the words listed above, so we do not need to consider them.

There is a limited number of wrong-answer options, but these options will be there in the answers to distract you. In the heat of the moment an answer may superficially look correct. So you need to read carefully the options and codes (i.e. perform "analysis").

CHAPTER 7

BMAT practice papers

SAMPLE PAPER A		With questions like these fill in the appropriate bubble with your chosen answer e.g.

SECTION 1A

Aptitude and Skills

Response Sheet

With questions like these fill in the appropriate bubble with your chosen answer e.g.

A B C D
○ ● ○ ○

With questions like these, write your answer clearly in the space provided with one letter or digit in each space. Use BLOCK CAPITALS

Name

Date Of Birth

`4` `3` . `2` `5`

1	A B C D	14	A B C D	27	
2	A B C D E	15	A B C D E	28	A B C D E
3	A B C D E	16	A B C D E	29	A B C D
4	A B C D E	17	A B C D	30	A B C D E
5	A B C D E	18	A B C D E	31	A B C D E
6	A B C D E	19	A B C D E	32	A B C D
7	A B C D	20	A B C D	33	A B C D
8	A B C D E	21	A B C D	34	
9	A B C D E	22	A B C D E	35	
10	A B C D E	23	A B C D		
11	A B C D	24	A B C D E		
12	A B C D E	25	A B C D E		
13	A B C D E	26	A B C D		

BMAT PRACTICE QUESTIONS

SAMPLE PAPER A

60 minutes

SECTION 1A   Aptitude and Skills

Instructions to Candidates

Please read this page carefully.

Speed as well as accuracy is important in this section. ***Work quickly, or you may not finish the paper.*** There are no penalties for incorrect responses, only points for correct answers, so you should attempt all 35 questions.

Unless otherwise stated, all questions are worth one mark.

Answer on the sheet provided. Many questions ask you to show your choice between options by shading a circle (or circles, if specified in the question).

Choose the option which best answers the question asked. If you make a mistake, erase it thoroughly and try again.

Calculators and dictionaries are NOT permitted.

1 It is 12 noon and the positions of the hour hand and the minute hand of the clock have just coincided. How long will it be before the two hands of the clock coincide again?

   A 3600 seconds
   B 3900 seconds
   C 3927 seconds
   D 4050 seconds

2 A bus leaves the station with a certain number of passengers. It drops half of its passengers at the first stop and a third of the remaining at the second stop. At the third stop one passenger gets out and a sixth the original number of passengers get on at the fourth stop. If there are two passengers left on the bus, what was the number of passengers on the bus when it left the station?

   A 2
   B 4
   C 6
   D 8
   E 12

3 **Argument**
   The superstores which are becoming ever more pervasive in society provide a one-stop shop for everyone's needs. Instead of visiting several different stores for food, clothes, electrical appliances, entertainment products, etc. these large out-of-town retailers save consumers time and often money, since larger stores have more buying power and hence can purchase cheaper stock and pass on these savings to customers. It is this desire of consumers for lower prices, without sacrificing quality, which is bankrupting smaller businesses, and causing the loss of local family-run shops. Many people lament the loss of these, but unless they match their sympathy with custom at the floundering establishments, the decline will continue.

   Statement
   Everyone who lives in a modern society must deal with the highly stressed, rushed-paced, hectic lifestyle where time is the major limiting factor.

   Which of the following best describes how the short statement relates to the argument?

   A Restates the main conclusion
   B Presents a serious challenge
   C Lends support
   D Paraphrases one of argument's main premises
   E It misses the point of the argument neither challenging nor supporting it

4 It takes a group of four bricklayers an hour to build a wall. How many minutes will it take the group to build the same wall, if two of them become injured so that the injured bricklayers can only work at one sixth the normal rate and the group is joined by one more fit bricklayer who works at the normal rate? (Assume all bricklayers work at the same normal rate.)

A 40
B 48
C 50
D 60
E 72

5 In an investigation of anti-cancer drugs it was found that the clearance of alemtuzumab was 80 mg/min greater than the clearance of epirubicin. Moreover, busulfan had a clearance of 200 mg/min while cyclophosphamide and dactinomycin had clearances of 240 mg/min and 180 mg/min, respectively. The mean clearance was determined to be 200 mg/min.

What was the clearance of alemtuzumab?

A 80 mg/min
B 130 mg/min
C 150 mg/min
D 230 mg/min
E 300 mg/min

6 The kidney produces urine by removing water and solutes from blood. Blood flows through the kidney of a certain mammal at a rate of 150 ml/min. The kidney removes all of a certain solute X dissolved in 20% of the blood that flows through it. If the volume of urine produced by this mammal is 21.6 litres over a 24-hour period and the concentration of solute X in the urine is 10 mg/ml what is the concentration of solute X in the mammal's blood?

A 1 mg/ml
B 2 mg/ml
C 3 mg/ml
D 5 mg/ml
E 10 mg/ml

7 Vegetarianism is certainly better for the environment than eating meat: every cow reared to provide beef for 1 person requires thirty acres of land whereas the same thirty acres of land could be used to grow maize or some other crop to feed 1200 people. Even without taking into account any other environmental factors, this shows that the environmental cost of eating meat is completely unjustifiable.

Which of the following if true most seriously weakens the above argument?

A Beef consumption has fallen in recent times due to the BSE crisis.

B Many vegetarians are not environmentally conscious.

C Non-meat animal produce, such as milk requires equivalent land use for animal rearing.

D A diet consisting of maize only is not as nutritious a one consisting of beef alone.

8 Carnivorous wild animals, such as tigers and other big cats possess a natural hunting instinct. They have acquired these primitive drives as essential survival adaptations over many thousands of years of evolution. Humans still have basic instincts, but there are also conditioning forces, which inhibit the expression of such instincts by virtue of humans' larger, more developed brains. To use big cats in circuses where they are "tamed" for entertainment purposes is sooner or later going to result in tragedy.

Which of the following best expresses the main conclusion of the argument?

A Big, wild cats are dangerous.

B It is impossible to completely suppress an animal's natural instincts.

C Humans are the only living organisms able to inhibit their natural instincts.

D Using wild animals for live entertainment is inherently dangerous.

E The differential ability of humans and animals to suppress their instincts is a sign of evolution.

9 Which **one** of the following statements is inconsistent with the others?

A The last egg released from a fish will have a greater mass than the first egg released.

B Eggs released at different times are located at different parts of the fish.

C The last egg released from a fish is the farthest from the tail fin.

D Eggs of the smallest mass are located farthest from a fish's tail fin.

E The first egg released from a fish will have a greater mass than the last egg released.

10 Selecting a student on the basis of ability is inevitable, if we are to maximise and not waste the educational potential of our young people. Some students are naturally inclined to pursue more academic careers whereas for others a vocational education is more desirable. Usually, this is apparent from a young age and should therefore be nurtured from that time. Without selection, students who are destined for either of these disciplines will be thwarted by an education system that attempts, in vain, to serve both groups. Those destined for an academic

career will feel unfulfilled whilst those destined for vocational jobs will feel that much of their time is being wasted, with very little in the way of vocational-skill training. Thus it seems obvious that students should be selected and separated on the basis of academic, technical and other specific abilities from a young age, with special emphasis given to these particular areas of talent in their future education.

Which two of the following if true would **seriously** weaken the above argument?

A The aptitudes and interests shown by students early on usually change with time.

B Vocational pursuits generally require some academic knowledge as well.

C The aptitudes most children demonstrate, rather than being inbuilt, are mainly directed by the type of education they receive.

D The process of selecting students at a young age may be psychologically damaging.

E Educational variety is important in building well balanced members of society.

11 Figure 1 shows the side view of a certain container. The vertical height of the liquid column in the container from the base is denoted by **h**. Figure 2 shows a representative cross section taken through the container at point z, while Figure 3 shows the rate at which the volume of liquid in the container and **h** change as it is being filled from empty.

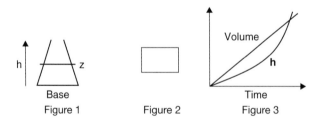

A second container shown below is to be filled with liquid.

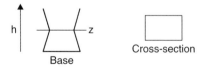

Which one of the following options best shows how both the rate at which the volume of liquid in the flask and **h** change as it is being filled with liquid from empty?

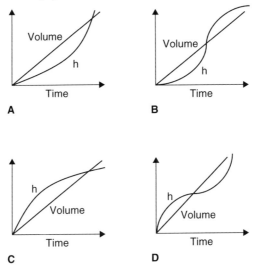

Questions 12 and 13 refer to the following information:

Each different letter below represents a specific digit. The calculations shown are accurate.

XE	X	X	FB
+ FB	+ E	× E	− XE
NBE	F	NX	WC

12 What digit does the letter E represent?

    A 2
    B 3
    C 4
    D 6
    E 8

13 Give the answer to the following sum:

        WC
      − XE
    ───────

    A FB
    B XB
    C XF
    D CE
    E DE

14 Many people enjoy cycling not only because it is a healthy way to exercise but also it is a non-polluting form of transport. Many European countries have excellent cycle networks in major towns and cities, where cycles even have priority over other vehicles. In the UK, with proper investment in national cycle routes to make cycling safer, the bicycle could replace the car for most journeys.

Which of the following best expresses the main flaw in the above argument?

A National cycle routes are not as extensive as road networks.
B It is impossible to transport heavy loads by bicycle hence this would not be suitable for industry.
C The fact that many people enjoy cycling does not mean they prefer cycling to travelling by car.
D The UK is one of the European countries where accidents involving cyclists is low.

15 The resentment felt in the West against major pharmaceutical companies for not selling anti-HIV drugs at cost price to developing countries is misplaced and uninformed. It does not take into account the massive investment required to produce a single drug, consider the many failures, which never reach the market or the capital required for future investment for further drug research and development. This investment comes from private shareholders who demand a profit on their investment. Since it takes a long time to recoup the costs of new drugs, let alone make a profit, these companies cannot be expected to lower the drug price in the developing world unless others, i.e. developed nations, which accounts for the major market, are prepared to pay higher prices for these drugs to offset this loss.

Which of the following if true will most seriously weaken the above argument?

A Pharmaceutical companies consistently make profits.
B Recent withdrawals of major drugs from the market demonstrate that companies cannot be assured of long-term income from individual drugs.
C Many shareholders are ready to make less of a profit for a social good.
D Drugs are usually on the market for longer than is necessary to recover costs.
E Western Governments are willing to subsidise pharmaceutical companies for selling drugs to developing countries at cost price.

16 When climbing a flight of 20 stairs Adam takes 2 steps back after every 5 steps forward. Using this method he needs to take a total of 40 steps to climb the 20 stairs. When climbing the same stairs Jonathan takes 2 steps back after every 3 steps forward but each of Jonathan's steps take half as long as Adam's.

What fraction of the time it took Adam to climb the stairs does it take Jonathan?

A 0.5
B 1.0
C 1.1
D 1.2
E 2.0

17 Phil is standing close to a mirror so that he can see both the time display in front of him and its reflection in the mirror. The diagram below shows an aerial view of Phil's head, the timer he is looking at and the mirror with the reflection of the timer.

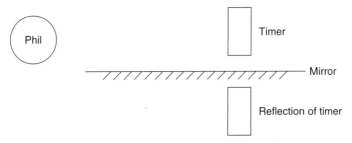

Below is what Phil sees on his timer and in the mirror when it is midnight.

Timer display	Reflection in mirror
00:00	*00:00*

Which of the following pairs is also possible?

	Timer display	Reflection in mirror
A	*12:12*	*15:51*
B	*13:57*	*15:31*
C	*09:45*	*24:20*
D	*08:06*	*60:80*

18 It must be indisputable that casinos and other forms of gambling ben-
    efit only the businesses and not the players. If these establishments paid
    more in winnings than they took in profit they would cease to trade.
    Therefore, although there is tiny minority of winners, who may take
    home a "large" jackpot, the vast majority consistently lose money.

    Which of the following is an implicit assumption of the above
    argument?

    A Casinos dupe players if necessary to make a profit.
    B Casino managers persuade successful players to continue gambling
       until they eventually lose.
    C Players who consistently lose money will not return in the future.
    D Casinos must make profit in order to be viable businesses.
    E Financial reward is the only benefit to be gained from gambling.

19 World oil production is about to reach a peak and then decline. Major
    oil companies are reporting drilling less oil than predicted across the
    world. America's oil production is already past its peak; indeed, increas-
    ing oil prices and new technology may help slow the inevitable but they
    cannot solve the problem. Recent discoveries are modest at best and
    even if the predictions of this decline are over-enthusiastic, it will come
    eventually since world oil reserves are finite. In view of the inability of
    current alternatives to fill the emerging vacuum, exploring alternative
    energy sources is now imperative – modern day civilisation cannot oth-
    erwise be sustained.

    Which of the following is an implicit assumption of the above
    argument?

    A The exploration and discovery of new oil reserves has ceased.
    B The pursuit by civilisation of a modern day lifestyle is a desirable and
       good thing.
    C New technologies such as hybrid cars are unlikely to help oil
       shortages.
    D The reliance on oil, the majority of which is imported, is politically
       unsafe.
    E Crude oil is too precious a commodity to burn in the internal com-
       bustion engine.

20 The power of suggestion can be very strong, but it cannot be used
    as a defence for wrongdoing. If one is told to do something illegal, it
    is always possible to resist depending on whether the will to resist is
    present in the first place. Similarly, if someone tells another person to
    perform an illegal act and he or she carries it out, it cannot be anyone's
    fault except the perpetrator of the act.

Which of the following best expresses the main conclusion of the above argument?

A Every person is wholly responsible for their actions.
B Most people are easily suggestible.
C Many people prefer wrongdoing.
D Individuals are generally responsible for acting on received suggestions.

Questions 21 to 24 refer to the following information:

The price of gold varies depending on the value of the currency being used to buy it and on local conditions. The relationship between supply and demand, for instance, has a strong impact on the price of gold; for example, an acute shortage of gold will cause an increase in gold prices whilst a reduced demand would cause the price to drop. The value or purchasing power of a currency follows the trend of local economic conditions.

Chart 1 below shows the trend in gold prices in terms of the currency of three countries: Byzantia (BZ), Iona (IO) and Sidon (SD).

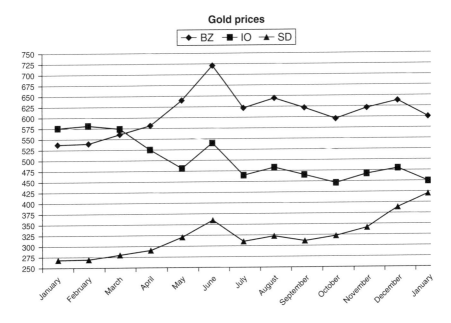

Chart 2 below shows the exchange rates between the different currencies over the same period. For example, in January, 1 BZ would be worth 0.75 IOs.

Chart 2	BZ→IO	IO→BZ	BZ→SD	SD→BZ	IO→SD	SD→IO
January	0.75000	1.33333	1.25000	0.80000	1.66667	0.60000
February	0.73000	1.36986	1.19048	0.84000	1.63079	0.61320
March	0.81000	1.23457	1.11111	0.90000	1.37174	0.72900
April	0.80000	1.25000	1.14943	0.87000	1.43678	0.69600
May	0.69000	1.44928	1.09890	0.91000	1.59261	0.62790
June	0.74000	1.35135	1.33333	0.75000	1.80180	0.55500
July	0.74000	1.35135	1.25000	0.80000	1.68919	0.59200
August	0.75000	1.33333	1.38889	0.72000	1.85185	0.54000
September	0.82000	1.21951	1.63934	0.61000	1.99920	0.50020
October	0.68000	1.47059	1.88679	0.53000	2.77469	0.36040
November	0.75000	1.33333	2.43902	0.41000	3.25203	0.30750
December	0.80000	1.25000	2.22222	0.45000	2.77778	0.36000
January	0.75000	1.33333	2.22222	0.45000	2.96296	0.33750

21 What was the average percentage change in gold price between June and December?

A 5

B 8

C 19

D 21

22 Which of the following would, without conflicting with the information given above, best explain the price of gold in IOs over the first 4 months?

A The value of IOs was relatively low over the first 4 months.

B Low purchasing power of the IO over the first 3 months was followed by a period of recovery in April and May.

C Government restrictions to gold imports in Iona officially ended in early April.

D Between March and June, Iona's goldmines started to wind down due to financial and labour constraints.

E The value of gold was higher in real terms over the first 4 months compared with the last 4 months.

23 Which of the following, if true, could possibly explain gold prices between May and mid-July?

(i) A worldwide shortage of gold.

(ii) Terrorist attacks affecting each of the goldmines of Byzantia, Iona and Sidon.

(iii) An increase in importation tax on gold in all three countries.

A i only   **C** i and iii only

B ii only   **D** i, ii and iii

24 Which of the following can most reliably be inferred about Sidon from the information given (assuming that local demand for gold in Sidon remained the same compared with the other two countries)?

   A Sidonese goldmines provide a ready supply of gold, allowing the price of gold to be relatively low.

   B The low price of gold in Sidon reflects the high purchasing power of its currency (the SD).

   C Sidon experienced an acute shortage of gold from November onwards.

   D An economic downturn from September finally affected local gold supply after a delay.

   E Over the year, the value of the SD has increased overall relative to IO and BZ.

25 There is no reason why marijuana should not be legalised. No one has ever died from smoking marijuana and legalising it will eliminate the need for an underground subculture: ready availability will decrease the marijuana-related crime rate. Moreover marijuana has medicinal values and has been proven to enhance creativity. It is also thought that marijuana creates pacifism and can act as a "stress reliever".

Based on the above paragraph, which of the following statements can be most reliably inferred?

   A A drug can be presumed to be safe if no one has died from taking it.

   B Overall marijuana is a beneficial drug.

   C Crime related to marijuana is a disadvantage of its prohibition.

   D The decision to legalise a drug is an important indicator of how many people die from its effects.

   E Marijuana should be used for medicinal purposes.

Questions 26 to 29 refer to the following information:

Jimmy's Car Dealership is facing an economic dilemma and the manager has decided to change the commission system by paying the luxury car salesmen a flat-rate commission of £800 for every car sold. This would replace the commission system, which all salesmen except luxury car salesmen still receive, of paying a fixed percentage of the sale. The manager decides that he may also need to fire one of his junior salesmen: either John (from the luxury car department) or Jeremy (from the small cars department) to save some more money. John is quick to point out that he makes more money for the company.

The table below shows John's and Jeremy's sales figures over a 6-month period after the commission structure is changed.

Month/year	John's sales			Jeremy's sales		
	Number of sales	Sales value (£)	Commission (£)	Number of sales	Sales value (£)	Commission (£)
May/08	6	99,402	4,800	8	100,536	5,027
June/08	8	124,536	6,400	12	125,244	6,262
July/08	6	111,402	4,800	14	122,710	6,136
August/08	7	129,969	5,600	10	96,760	4,838
September/08	8	164,536	6,400	7	78,638	3,932
October/08	8	156,536	6,400	6	75,384	3,769
Total	43	786,381	34,400	57	599,272	29,964

26 What is the difference between the average prices of a car sold by Jeremy compared with a car sold by John within the 6-month period?

   A £525
   B £800
   C £7,450
   D £7,775

27 How much has the manager saved from John in the 6-month period by changing the commission structure? (Give your answer to the nearest £10.)

28 What would be the additional savings if the same commission system used for luxury car salesmen were also used for Jeremy (paying £500 per car sold)?

   A £1,464
   B £3,456
   C £6,384
   D £6,900
   E £8,464

29 Each shape in the table below represents a specific number. The numbers in the table shows the sum of the shapes along each row and column.

Which of the following options shows the shapes arranged in descending order of magnitude from left to right?

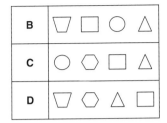

Questions 30 and 31 refer to the following information:

Three men – Andrew, Harry and Phil – and three women – Sandy, Rosie and Mary – all go camping to Hawaii where they live in tents. There are ten tents arranged in two rows of five each. Each tent directly faces a tent in the other row. Andrew and Phil live in tents at the opposite ends of the same row. Andrew lives in two tents which are side by side on the same row. Sandy and Rosie live next to each other on the same row. Mary lives in the central tent on the same row as Andrew and Harry and there is a vacant tent across from her. Rosie lives next to a vacant tent and Sandy lives at the end of the row.

30 Who lives across from Sandy?

    A Andrew
    B Harry
    C Phil
    D Andrew or Phil
    E Andrew or Harry

31 How many people live on Sandy's row?

    A 2
    B 3
    C 4
    D 2 or 3
    E 2 or 3 or 4

Questions 32 to 35 refer to the following information:

The Chinese one child policy is unique in the history of the world. It was a source of great pain for one generation, but a generation later it began to yield important economic benefits. For China, and the world as a whole, the one child policy was one of the most important social policies ever implemented.

Rapid population growth is an unforgiving taskmaster. Even with the one child policy – as a result of the high birth rate a generation before – China still has one million more births than deaths every 5 weeks. The Chinese

State Council launched the policy in 1979. Could China ever have achieved the same results without the one child policy? Possibly. Between 1952 and 1979, the Chinese total fertility rate fell from 6.5 to 2.75, and today all age groups and social classes prefer to have two children or fewer. Some western commentators believe China over-reacted, whereas others emphasise that even small changes in the timing of a decline in fertility are important. The difference between a total fertility rate of 2.1, which might have been achieved without the policy, and a total fertility rate of 1.6 (found today) releases 24% more resources for the family and national investment. The Indian economy has begun to grow rapidly, but unlike China the decline in fertility has been uneven, and states such as Bihar and Uttar Pradesh (total fertility rates of 4.4 and 4.8) remain mired in poverty.

Undoubtedly, the one child policy caused great individual pain and it has been heavily criticised. For people in the US especially, the idea that society's long-term interests could ever be more important than individual rights was anathema. A veritable media industry has arisen in the US criticising the one child policy, although it chooses to overlook the tens of millions of coercive pregnancies in other countries where family planning and legal abortion are not available. The US administration refuses to fund the United Nations Population Fund because it works in China, even though this fund has never supported the one child policy.

Potts, M – *British Medical Journal* 333; 361–362.

32 Which one of the following can least reliably be inferred from the passage?

  A China's one child policy is exceptional.
  B Rapid population growth is a bad thing.
  C It is possible that China would have achieved the current level of growth without the one child policy.
  D Implementation of the one child policy was a difficult experience for the Chinese people.

33 According to the passage which of the following best explains why a falling birth rate may be economically beneficial?

  A A falling birth rate means a smaller population and so lower consumption of resources.
  B A falling birth rate means less time for frivolities such as sex and more time for economically productive work.
  C A falling birth rate means fewer people dependent on state benefits.
  D A falling birth rate means fewer children generally and a relative increase in the working age group of the population.

34 If the current population of China is 1.8 billion, what is China's current annual growth rate? (Give your answer as a percentage to the nearest one decimal place.)

35 According to the passage, "the difference between a total fertility rate of 2.1, which might have been achieved without the policy and a total fertility rate of 1.6 (found today) releases 24% more resources for the family and national investment."

How much more resources (rather than 24%) would have been released if the fertility rate "found today" was to be 1.9 instead of 1.6? (Give your answer as a percentage to the nearest percent.)

END OF SECTION 1

SAMPLE PAPER A

SECTION 2A Scientific Knowledge and Application

Response Sheet

With questions like these fill in the appropriate bubble with your chosen answer e.g.

A B C D
○ ● ○ ○

With questions like these, write your answer clearly in the space provided with one letter or digit in each space. Use BLOCK CAPITALS

| 4 | 3 | . | 2 | 5 |

Name

Date Of Birth

1   A B C D E
    ○ ○ ○ ○ ○

2   ☐☐☐☐☐☐

3   a ☐☐☐☐☐
    b ☐☐☐☐☐

4   A B C D E
    ○ ○ ○ ○ ○

5   A B C D E
    ○ ○ ○ ○ ○

6   ☐☐☐☐☐☐

7   A B C D
    ○ ○ ○ ○

8   a ☐☐☐☐☐
    b ☐☐☐☐☐

9   i ☐ ii ☐ iii ☐

10 i ☐ ii ☐ iii ☐ iv ☐

11 i ☐ ii ☐ iii ☐
    iv ☐ v ☐

12 A B C D E
    ○ ○ ○ ○ ○

13 A B C D E
    ○ ○ ○ ○ ○

14 A B C D E
    ○ ○ ○ ○ ○

15 A B C D
    ○ ○ ○ ○

16 A B C D
    ○ ○ ○ ○

17 ☐☐☐ : ☐☐☐

18 ☐☐☐☐☐☐

19 ☐☐☐☐☐☐

20 A B C D E
    ○ ○ ○ ○ ○

21 a ☐ b ☐
    c ☐ d ☐

22 A B C D E
    ○ ○ ○ ○ ○

23 A B C D
    ○ ○ ○ ○

24 i ☐ ii ☐ iii ☐

25 A B C D E
    ○ ○ ○ ○ ○

26 A B C D E
    ○ ○ ○ ○ ○

27 A B C D E
    ○ ○ ○ ○ ○

30 minutes

SECTION 2A   Scientific Knowledge and Application

Instructions to Candidates

Please read this page carefully. Speed as well as accuracy is important in this section. *Work quickly, or you may not finish the paper*. There are no penalties for incorrect responses, only points for correct answers, so you should attempt all 27 questions.

Unless otherwise stated, all questions are worth one mark.

Answer on the sheet provided. Many questions ask you to show your choice between options by shading a circle (or circles, if specified in the question).

If questions ask you to write in words or numbers be sure to write clearly in the spaces provided.

Choose the option which best answers the question asked. If you make a mistake, erase it thoroughly and try again.

Calculators are NOT permitted.

1 In the diagram below, a bag made of a semi-permeable membrane material (M) is suspended in a tank. The bag and the tank are filled with two different solutions (A and B).

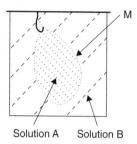

Solution A   Solution B

If solution A is 10% glucose and solution B is 25% glucose which of the following statements are true:

A Water diffuses from the tank into the bag.
B Glucose moves from the tank into the bag.
C Glucose is broken down in the tank and stored inside the bag.
D Water moves by osmosis from the bag into the tank.
E Glucose moves by osmosis from bag into the tank.

2 Calculate the area bounded by the equations: $y = 15 - 3x$ and $y/3 + 4 = 2x$ and the **x-axis**.

3 An object made entirely from one material has a volume of $30\,m^3$. It floats in a liquid of density $3\,g/cm^3$ with only half its mass below the liquid's surface. The object is then placed in another liquid of the same volume but with a density of $1\,g/cm^3$. If the final upthrust that will act on the object is expressed in the form $a \times 10^b\,N$ give the values of a and b. (Assume $g = 10\,m/s^2$)

4 Carbon dioxide reacts with water in the blood to form carbonic acid, H_2CO_3. This is likely to have a pH of approximately:

A 0
B 2.5
C 5.5
D 7.5
E 12.5

5 The gene causing cystic fibrosis, CFTR, is inherited in an autosomal recessive manner. A group of 20 carriers of the CFTR gene and their partners who are also all carriers of the same gene is followed up for a research study. Between them they have 45 children. A carrier does not suffer from cystic fibrosis. Approximately how many of these children would you expect to suffer from cystic fibrosis?

A 2   **B** 5   **C** 12   **D** 24   **E** 45

6 The mass of a hydrogen atom is approximately 1.67×10^{-24}g while that of a uranium atom is approximately 3.95×10^{-22}g.

   How many times heavier is a uranium atom than a hydrogen molecule? Give your answer to three significant figures.

7 Which of the following graphs best illustrates the relationship between power and current for a given ohmic resistor?

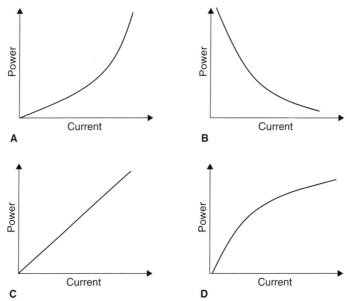

8 Solve the equation $x^2 - 4x = 7$. Give your answer in the form $x = a \pm \sqrt{b}$.

9 Below shows a system which maintains calcium homoeostasis. Without the system, calcium levels in the blood tend to decrease. Calcium levels in the blood are controlled by a negative feedback mechanism. Low levels of free (unbound) calcium are sensed by the parathyroid gland, causing its activity to increase and release parathyroid hormone, which stimulates the release of calcium from bone. Calcium bound to protein in the blood is in equilibrium with free calcium. Together they make up the total calcium in the blood.

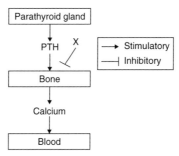

Select the correct option (**A** to **F**) from the table below which best represents what would initially happen in the following scenarios:

(**i**)   Injection of substance X (an irreversible antagonist of PTH).
(**ii**)   Addition of a binding resin that binds free calcium.
(**iii**) Continuous injection of additional PTH into the blood.

	Total calcium in blood	Free calcium in blood	PTH	Parathyroid activity	Bone
A	Increase	Increase	Increase	Decrease	Net breakdown
B	Increase	No change	Increase	Decrease	Net breakdown
C	No change	Decrease	Increase	Increase	Net breakdown
D	No change	Decrease	No change	No change	No change
E	Decrease	Decrease	Increase	Increase	No change
F	Decrease	Decrease	Increase	Increase	Net breakdown

10 The diagram below shows the apparatus used for the electrolysis of aqueous sodium chloride. Match the correct word or term (labelled **A** to **F**) from the list below with the apparatus components (**i** to **ii**) and gaseous products (**iii** to **iv**) on the diagram.

A anode
B cathode
C chlorine
D electrolyte
E hydrogen
F oxygen

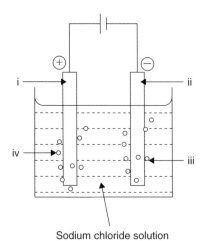

Sodium chloride solution

11 The table below shows the gaseous composition and temperature of air and blood at different locations (**A** to **E**) in a healthy human body.

	A	B	C	D	E
O_2 (%)	21	16	20	18	15
CO_2 (%)	0.04	4	0.04	1	4.2
N_2 (%)	78	76	78	77	78
H_2O (%)	1.3	6.2	100	100	100
Temperature (°C)	20	37	37	37	37

Using the information above, match each of the following named locations with the correct corresponding column (**A** to **E**) from the table above. Each option may be used only once.

(i)   Coronary (heart) artery
(ii) Hepatic (liver) venule
(iii) Skin capillary
(iv) Inspired air (in mouth)
(v)   Exhaled air (in trachea)

12 The circuit below shows a 24 V battery and three resistors. What is the current in the 6 ohms resistor?

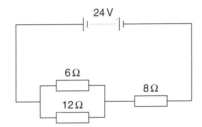

A 0.75 A
B 1.3 A
C 2 A
D 3 A
E 4 A

13 The graphs below show the temperature changes seen when a solid is heated (left) and a gas is cooled (right).

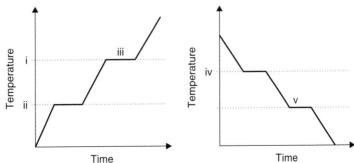

Which option (**A** to **E**) correctly identifies the labels on the graphs (**i** to **v**)?

	i	ii	iii	iv	v
A	Melting point	Boiling point	Condensing	Freezing point	Melting
B	Melting point	Boiling point	Freezing	Melting point	Freezing
C	Boiling point	Freezing point	Boiling	Melting point	Boiling
D	Boiling point	Melting point	Boiling	Boiling point	Freezing
E	Freezing point	Melting Point	Melting	Boiling point	Condensing

14 Which of the following options exhibits the greatest amount of energy? (Assume $g = 10\,\text{m/s}^2$)

A An electrical load of 12 ohms with a current of 4 A running through it.
B A mass of 30 kg moving at a speed of 3 m/s.
C A 10 kg ball, 1 m above the ground.
D Pulling a stone of mass 13 kg along the ground for 1.5 m (Friction = 0 N).

15 A certain insect toxin attacks plant cells, inhibiting photosynthesis. What are the chemical changes in the plant cell likely to be?

A A fall in glucose and an increase in lactic acid.
B Glucose decreases and carbon dioxide increases.
C Carbon dioxide decreases and glucose decreases.
D Oxygen, glucose and carbon dioxide stay the same, and water decreases.

16 Assuming the equations given below are correct which of the options (**A** to **D**) is a possibility?

	Equation	Number and type of radiation emitted in conversion of X to Y
A	$^{238}_{92}\text{X} \longrightarrow \ ^{230}_{90}\text{Y}$	2 α particles and 2 γ rays
B	$^{238}_{92}\text{X} \longrightarrow \ ^{240}_{92}\text{Y}$	2 β particles and 2 γ rays
C	$^{238}_{92}\text{X} \longrightarrow \ ^{230}_{91}\text{Y}$	2 α particles, 3 β particles and 2 γ rays
D	$^{238}_{92}\text{X} \longrightarrow \ ^{238}_{90}\text{Y}$	2 γ rays

17 In a chemical process, a particular tungsten hydride is found to contain 0.92 kg of tungsten (W) and 0.015 kg of hydrogen (H). What is the tungsten to hydrogen ratio of this compound?

Relative atomic masses: W = 184; H = 1

Questions 18 and 19 refer to the information below:

The angles of elevation and depression of the top and base of an arrow as seen by a viewer's eye are 9° and 6° respectively, as shown in the diagram below. PR = 5 m.

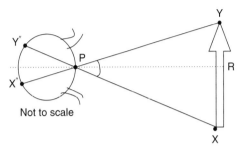

Not to scale

18 Assuming PR is perpendicular to XY calculate the length of XY in metres. Use the table below as appropriate.

Angle x	1	2	3	4	5	6	7	8	9	10	11
sin x	0.0174	0.0349	0.0523	0.0698	0.0872	0.1045	0.1219	0.1392	0.1564	0.1736	0.1908
cos x	0.9998	0.9994	0.9986	0.9976	0.9962	0.9945	0.9925	0.9903	0.9877	0.9848	0.9816
tan x	0.0175	0.0349	0.0524	0.0699	0.0875	0.1051	0.1228	0.1405	0.1584	0.1763	0.1944

19 If the distance to the back of the eye is 0.025 m, and assuming the eye is a regular circle, calculate the size of the image projected onto the back of the eye (X″Y″).

20 An atrial septal defect is an abnormal connection between the right atrium and left atrium of the heart. In someone with an atrial septal defect, compared with an equivalent normal person, there will be:

A More deoxygenated blood in the right atrium
B Less oxygenated blood in the lungs
C More oxygenated blood in the left atrium
D Less oxygenated blood in the rest of the body
E Less deoxygenated blood in the left ventricle

21 The reaction of ammonia and oxygen in the first step of the production of nitric acid is shown below:

Equation 1: $\mathbf{a}NH_3$ (g) + $\mathbf{b}O_2$ (g) → $\mathbf{c}NO$ (g) + $\mathbf{d}H_2O$ (I)

Balance the equation, giving whole number values for **a**, **b**, **c** and **d**.

22 The device shown below is used to lift an object of mass 100 kg from rest to 50 m/s in 10 seconds in the absence of any air resistance. To do this an evenly spread force of 50 N is applied to the whole of piston A. What is the ratio of area of piston B to the area of piston A? (Assume $g = 10 \text{ m/s}^2$)

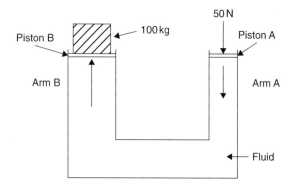

A 10
B 12
C 15
D 20
E 25

23 Which of the following values of x completely satisfy the following inequality?

$$x^2 \leqslant 18 - 3x$$

A $-4, -5, 7, 8$
B $-3, -4, -5, -7$
C $-2, -1, 2, 4$
D $6, 7, 8, 9$

24 A diabetic patient and a non-diabetic control subject both drink a solution of glucose at the point marked G on the graph. Two hours later they are injected with one of the following solutions:

Solution X: distilled water
Solution Y: insulin
Solution Z: insulin and protease (incubated at 37°C for 5 hours)

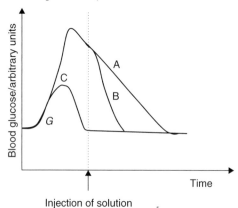

Which graph (**A** to **C**) best represents:

(i) The control subject taking *solution X*
(ii) The diabetic patient taking *solution Y*
(iii) The diabetic patient taking *solution Z*

25 What is the energy exerted when a boy pushes a 12 kg box along the ground in a straight line for 4 m if the average friction acting between the box and the ground is 70 N? (Assume $g = 10\,\text{ms}^2$)

A 280 J   **D** 760 J
B 336 J   **E** 840 J
C 480 J

26 The alkanes are hydrocarbons with the general formula C_nH_{2n+2}. Pentane (C_5H_{12}) has three isomers, which are shown below as Isomer A, B and C.

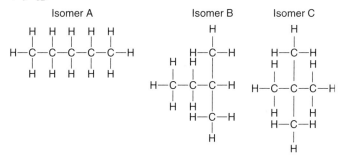

Which one of the following properties of Isomer C, compared to the equivalent property in Isomer A, is correct?

A It has stronger intermolecular forces
B It is more unsaturated
C It has a lower boiling point
D It is heavier
E None of the above

27 The following is a schematic of the electromagnetic spectrum. **X** represents visible light, with **Y** and **Z** corresponding to red and blue light respectively.

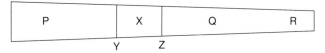

Which one of the following options (**A** to **E**) is correct?

A The frequency of **P** is higher than that of **R**
B The speed of **Q** is faster than the speed of **P**
C The frequency of **Y** is greater than that of **Z**
D The wavelength of **R** is shorter than that of **P**
E Gamma radiation has a longer wavelength than radio waves

END OF SECTION 2

30 minutes

SECTION 3A Writing Task

Instructions to Candidates

This question paper contains a choice of three tasks, of which you must answer only **one**. It also provides space in which you may make any preliminary notes you wish, but your answer must be written on a single page of an A4 sheet.

The tasks each provide an opportunity for you to show how well you can:

- select, develop and organise ideas and
- communicate them effectively in writing.

Before you begin writing, think carefully about what you need to say and the ways in which the organisation and layout of your response might help convey your message, diagrams, etc. may be used if they enhance communication.

Take care to show how well you can write and be concise, clear and accurate.

Dictionaries may *not* be used.

Remember that when you are told that you may begin you will have only 30 minutes to choose and complete your task, and that your complete response must be contained on a single side of an A4 sheet. The disciplines involved in this are regarded as key features of the task.

YOU MUST ANSWER ONLY <u>ONE</u> OF THE FOLLOWING QUESTIONS

1 **Experience must be our only guide, reason may mislead us.**
John Dickinson, American Constitutional Congress

Write a unified essay in which you address the following:

This is a statement concerning knowledge in general; explain what you think it means. Advance a counter-argument: that reason must be our only guide.

2 **The failure of scientific development to take the masses along with it, in the 21st century more than ever, will limit the application of scientific research and the range of scientific enquiry permitted in the near future.**

Write a unified essay in which you address the following:

What do you think this statement means and why do you think the author holds this viewpoint? Do you think this "failure" can be rectified? If so how?

3 **The concepts of merit and equality are incompatible; to have one you must jettison the other.**

Write a unified essay in which you address the following:

What do you think the statement means? Put forward an argument supporting the statement. Advance an argument against this conclusion, i.e. that merit and equality are compatible.

END OF SECTION 3

END OF PAPER 1

SAMPLE PAPER B

SECTION 1B   **Aptitude and Skills**

Response Sheet

With questions like these fill in the appropriate bubble with your chosen answer e.g.

A B C D
○ ● ○ ○

With questions like these, write your answer clearly in the space provided with one letter or digit in each space.
Use BLOCK CAPITALS

| 4 | 3 | . | 2 | 5 |

Name

Date Of Birth

1   A B C D
    ○ ○ ○ ○

2   A B C D E
    ○ ○ ○ ○ ○

3   A B C D E
    ○ ○ ○ ○ ○

4   A B C D E F
    ○ ○ ○ ○ ○ ○

5   A B C D E
    ○ ○ ○ ○ ○

6   A B C D
    ○ ○ ○ ○

7   A B C D
    ○ ○ ○ ○

8   A B C D E
    ○ ○ ○ ○ ○

9   A B C D E
    ○ ○ ○ ○ ○

10 A B C D E
    ○ ○ ○ ○ ○

11 A B C D E
    ○ ○ ○ ○ ○

12 A B C D E
    ○ ○ ○ ○ ○

13 A B C D E
    ○ ○ ○ ○ ○

14 A B C D E
    ○ ○ ○ ○ ○

15 A B C D
    ○ ○ ○ ○

16 A B C D E
    ○ ○ ○ ○ ○

17 A B C D E
    ○ ○ ○ ○ ○

18 A B C D E F
    ○ ○ ○ ○ ○ ○

19 A B C D E
    ○ ○ ○ ○ ○

20 A B C D E
    ○ ○ ○ ○ ○

21 A B C D
    ○ ○ ○ ○

22 A B C D E
    ○ ○ ○ ○ ○

23 A B C D E
    ○ ○ ○ ○ ○

24 □□□□□□

25 A B C D
    ○ ○ ○ ○

26 A B C D
    ○ ○ ○ ○

27 A B C D E
    ○ ○ ○ ○ ○

28 □ : □ : □

29 A B C D E
    ○ ○ ○ ○ ○

30 A B C D E
    ○ ○ ○ ○ ○

31 A B C D E
    ○ ○ ○ ○ ○

32 A B C D E
    ○ ○ ○ ○ ○

33 A B C D E
    ○ ○ ○ ○ ○

34 A B C D E
    ○ ○ ○ ○ ○

35 A B C D
    ○ ○ ○ ○

BMAT PRACTICE QUESTIONS

SAMPLE PAPER B

Paper 1B   60 minutes

SECTION 1   Aptitude and Skills

Instructions to Candidates

Please read this page carefully.

Speed as well as accuracy is important in this section. ***Work quickly, or you may not finish the paper.*** There are no penalties for incorrect responses, only points for correct answers, so you should attempt all 35 questions.

Unless otherwise stated, all questions are worth one mark.

Answer on the sheet provided. Many questions ask you to show your choice between options by shading a circle (or circles, if specified in the question).

Choose the option which best answers the question asked. If you make a mistake, erase it thoroughly and try again.

Calculators and dictionaries are *not* permitted.

1 The emergence of potentially dangerous products from civilian (non-military) genetic engineering laboratories is now more likely than ever. Not only is the field of genetics at its most active but the less than stringent protocols applied by committees responsible for vetting research proposals have not helped the situation. A greater problem exists in that academics on the whole choose to ignore the potential threats for fear of an indiscriminate backlash against the science of biotechnology. In order to counter this problem, by law PhD degrees in the field should only be awarded to students who can show how their work might contribute to the development of biological weapons. Such a radical legislation will alter the current attitude which provides very little to stand in the way of a potential disaster.

Which of the following best summarises the main conclusion of the above argument?

A The prevailing attitude of self-preservation by academics has resulted in the increased potential danger from genetic engineering laboratories.
B Genetic engineering provides an inexorable route to disaster because of the likelihood of producing dangerous products.
C PhD students must be forced to show how their work might contribute to the development of biological weapons.
D The world of bio-engineering is awash with the risks of bio-terrorism.

2 A car leaves Cincinnati for Dayton on the same 100 km road as a motorbike that leaves Dayton for Cincinnati. Both vehicles set out simultaneously at 12:45. The motorbike travels at a speed 100 km/h in excess of the car. They cross paths at 13:05. What is the speed of the car?

A 50 km/h
B 80 km/h
C 100 km/h
D 120 km/h
E 150 km/h

3 Two wheels A and B each have a black marking on a specific point along their circumference. The circumference of wheel A is 24 m while that of wheel B is 15 m. Wheel A and wheel B are moved along the ground at rates of 2 m/s and 3 m/s, respectively and the black markings on both wheels have just touched the ground at this moment for the first time. What further distance will wheel B have covered by the time the black marking on both wheels simultaneously touch the ground for the fourth time?

A 60 m
B 120 m
C 180 m
D 540 m
E 720 m

4 The Government Transport Department recently finished a 3-year study into the effectiveness of speed cameras in saving lives. They found that the benefits to society in avoided injuries and other savings came to £220 million, while the cameras cost only £54 million to run. Over the 3 years studied, there was a 40% reduction in accidents at camera sites. The vast majority of people surveyed support speed camera use and think that they do work and are necessary.

Which **two** of the following if true would most seriously weaken the above argument?

A If drivers are constantly monitoring their speedometer they are less likely to be paying attention on driving and more likely to have accidents.

B The 3-year study did not take into account safety measures other than speed cameras at the sites of camera installation.

C Most accidents are caused by non-speeding drivers who are otherwise unfit to drive, e.g. under the influence of drugs.

D Low speed driving is more monotonous than high speed driving so drivers are less likely to fall asleep and have accidents while driving at high speed.

E Driving to the speed limit has increased journey times and therefore the time exposed to accident risk.

F Accidents overall may have decreased but the number of fatal accidents has increased.

5 All brown things are bears. All furry things are scary and all scary things are fuzzy. If I am white and fuzzy and the preceding assumptions are accurate, which of the following statements must be true?

A I am not a bear

B I am not a scary bear

C I am a furry bear

D I am definitely scary but not a bear

E I am not necessarily scary but I might be a bear

6 Two jugs A and B are filled to capacity with tea. Jug A holds 60 cups more than jug B. If 10 cups of tea were to be taken from each jug, jug A would then contain 3 times as much tea as jug B. What is the combined total number of cups of tea in the two full jugs?

A 120

B 140

C 150

D 210

7 The graphs below show the predicted and actual financial results for end of year profits from 1990 to 2005 for a certain retailer.

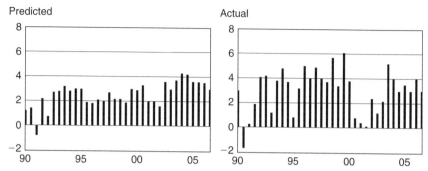

Which of the following accurately shows the difference between predicted results and actual results? (For each graph, positive readings represent a prediction that was above actual; negative readings represent a prediction that was below.)

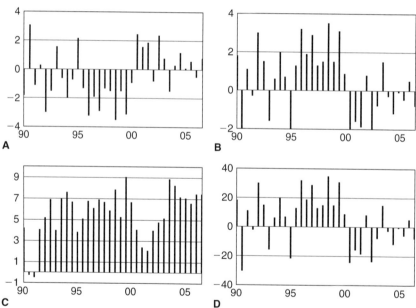

8 My last salary was 5% less than my current salary and my current salary is 25% more than my friend's salary. By what percentage is my last salary greater than my friend's salary?

    A 15.87%
    B 18.75%
    C 20%
    D 21%
    E 26.67%

9 The death penalty is, at best, no more of a deterrent than a sentence of life in prison. In fact, some criminologists maintain that the death penalty has the opposite effect: that is, society is brutalised by the use of the death penalty, and this increases the likelihood of more murder. States in the US that do not employ the death penalty generally have lower murder rates than states that do. The same is true when the US is compared to countries similar to it. The US, with the death penalty, has a higher murder rate than the countries of Europe or Canada, which do not use the death penalty.

Which of the following if true best supports the above argument?

A The death penalty for murder and such grave offences is essential to maintain a sense of justice in society.

B Most death row convicts have their death penalty sentence revoked before they are executed.

C Most people who commit murder either do not expect to get caught or do not weigh the consequences of their actions.

D Murder rates in the US cannot be reliably compared to murder rates in European countries because of less gun crime in Europe.

E Many people with criminal tendencies are indifferent to life in prison or the death penalty.

10 Recent news reported a vaccine for cervical cancer is now widely available. The science behind this innovation is that two viruses – human papilloma virus (HPV) 16 and 18 – are responsible for over 95% of cervical cancer. These viruses are spread through sexual contact. However, to see any benefit, all girls (and perhaps boys too) would need to be vaccinated before they became sexually active, to prevent spread of this virus. Some commentators are concerned however that vaccinating children against what is in essence a sexually transmitted disease will encourage youngsters to have more sex, and with that all the adverse social consequences which this entails.

Which one of the following if true would seriously weaken the argument of "some commentators"?

A Most children who are currently vaccinated do not understand what they are being vaccinated against.

B Young people do not base their decision on when to have sex on the likelihood of contracting a sexually transmitted disease.

C The UK already has the highest rate of underage sex and teenage pregnancy in Europe.

D Most cases of HPV are transmitted in adulthood.

E Cervical cancer rates have fallen where HPV vaccines have been introduced.

11 The table below shows the constitution of the Senate by party and by profession both at the beginning and at the end of session.

		Members of the Senate	
		Beginning of session	End of session
Party	Liberals	48	63
	Conservatives	52	57
Profession	Lawyers	60	60
	Doctors	40	40
	Engineers	0	8
	Managers	0	11
	Housewives	0	1

At the end of session the number of Conservatives who are not Doctors is 47 and the number of Liberal Engineers is greater than the number of Liberal Managers. If the number of Liberal Lawyers is 24 and the Housewife is a Liberal, what is the minimum possible number of Conservative Managers in the Senate at the end of the session?

A 2

B 3

C 5

D 6

E 8

12 A study has claimed to show that abnormal blood levels of prostate specific antigen (PSA) may be an indicator of prostate cancer. Twenty per cent of men with prostate cancer have normal PSA levels and at least 2 out of 3 men with abnormal PSA levels do not have prostate cancer. Tests were performed on a group of 2,500 men and 1,051 of them had normal blood PSA levels. What is the maximum possible number of men you would expect to have prostate cancer?

A 200

B 241

C 483

D 604

E 724

13 Gemma had a dog that initially cost her £200/month to maintain. She then adopted a new plan which cut her costs by 10% for the first month of use and by a further 15% for the second month of use. How much did Gemma save cumulatively over the 2 months by using this new plan?

A £20

B £47

C £50

D £67

E £77

14 The velocity of a car is the rate at which the car moves in a *particular direction from* a certain point in a straight line. Velocity becomes negative whenever the car is moving in the opposite direction, i.e. in the direction towards the point in question.

The graph below shows how the velocity from point 1 of a moving car varies over time for a particular journey. Point 2 denotes the point at which the car is at the farthest distance from point 1.

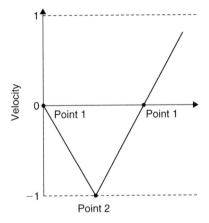

The acceleration of a car is the rate at which its velocity changes with time.

The graph below shows how the acceleration of another moving car varies with time for a particular journey

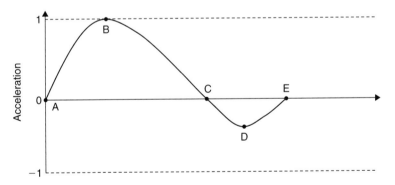

At what point (**A** to **E**) on the graph does the car have maximum velocity?

15 The theory behind the use of ID cards seems reasonable enough. The idea that it will help fight crime such as tax evasion, welfare fraud and terrorist activity as well as increasing police powers is indeed compelling in an age where information is as potent a weapon as any conventional

police tactic. Proponents of ID cards have added that their use could be voluntary rather than compulsory and add further that they would help all carriers by enabling more efficient receipt of government services. However, it is merely an impractical and fundamentally flawed tool, not to mention its high cost of implementation. ID cards would simply add further burden to law-abiding citizens whilst technology-savvy criminals escape through the inevitable loopholes. In order for ID cards to be effective in their primary purpose, they would have to be universal. The only way to make them universal is to make them compulsory. The inevitable fines and other types of punishment that will result (for those who do not comply) will only worsen matters.

Which one or more of the options below reliably follows from the above?

A If it can be ensured that ID cards are universal, they will be able to serve their primary purpose.
B ID cards are generally a good and welcome idea.
C Compulsory requirements must be backed by punishment for offenders.
D The use of ID cards cannot be voluntary.

16 Global warming is a major concern to most scientists, yet political action has not responded in the same way. Many industrialised nations fear that capping carbon emissions will harm their powerful economies and increase unemployment. Developing countries believe it is against their interests to stop burning cheap and readily available fossil fuels to build up their economies, in the same way the industrialised countries did before them.

What is the underlying assumption of the developing countries?

A No cheaper alternative energy sources exist.
B Present day industrialised countries have an advantage over them.
C Fossil fuels are in ready supply.
D They will not harm their countries by using fossil fuels.
E Capping carbon emissions is impossible.

17 When I start my computer different coloured dots move across my computer screen from the left edge to the right edge at different speeds. They always emerge from the left edge again in the same order and at the same rate they exited from the right edge. Assume that they start out together at the same time from the left edge of the screen when I switch my computer on. The red and green dots move at twice and a third the speed of the yellow and blue dots, respectively, while the red dot moves at a quarter the speed of the blue dot.

How many times would the green dot have moved across the full length of my screen by the first time all the dots coincide?

A 6
B 8
C 12
D 24
E 48

Questions 18 to 20 refer to the information below:

Moby's manufacturing, a producer and seller of car-engine parts undertakes a sales review of six products modified at the beginning of the year. All items are sold in standard quantities and packaging, known as "units", with each unit sold at a fixed price, known as the "unit price". The sales figures relating to each product are those gained from all units of that product sold over a given time period. A graph showing the sales figures are shown below.

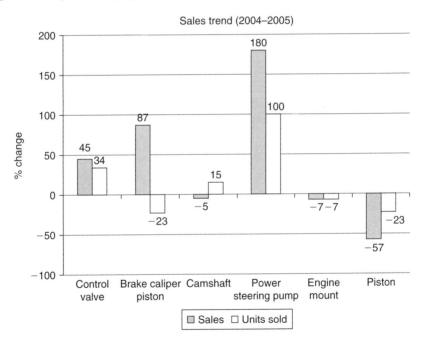

Sales trend (2004–2005)

18 Which product(s) have shown a reduction in unit price from 2004 to 2005?

A Control valve
B Brake calliper piston
C Camshaft
D Power steering pump
E Engine mount
F Piston

19 Which of the following can most reliably be concluded about the sales of modified products in the year shown?

A The modifications have been profitable since overall sales have increased.

B Overall, sales of the modified products are lower than last year (before they were modified).

C On average, there has been a 33% increase in the number of units sold.

D Overall, the percentage increase in sales has exceeded the increase in unit price.

E Of all the products the pistons have shown the lowest change in sales this year.

20 Which of the following shows the smallest change in unit price that would help improve sales to pre-modification levels when applied separately to both the engine mounts and pistons (assuming other factors remain the same)?

A 12% increase

B 58% increase

C 70% increase

D 160% increase

E 235% increase

21 A small business may be defined by the number of people it employs or by the amount of turnover per year. On the whole small businesses inject more into the economy than large businesses and there are far more small businesses in the country than large businesses which typically turn over a lot more annually individually. Therefore, entrepreneurship should be promoted by the government to improve the economy. Lower taxation would be an incentive to encourage business persons to run small businesses; another would be non-repayable loans available to business start-ups.

Which one or more of the following is an implicit assumption of the above argument?

A There are more people employed by small businesses overall than large ones.

B Improving the nation's economy is a priority of the government.

C Entrepreneurship usually involves small businesses.

D Small businesses, when taken individually, always employ fewer people than large businesses.

22 Below are translations of sentences from the ancient language of Noomoo:

Lon-ton-pop: You were late today
Jon-san-pop: You will come tomorrow

Shon-sin-mop: I came yesterday
Shock-sin-hop: She came last week

Assuming a conserved word order, which of the following means, "I will run tomorrow"?

A Shon-xan-pop
B Jon-san-mop
C Shon-xon-pop
D Jon-can-mop
E Sin-pop-can

Questions 23 to 25 refer to the information below:

The following graph shows the number of deaths from all causes in the world for developing and developed countries and for the age groups 0–4 and 5+.

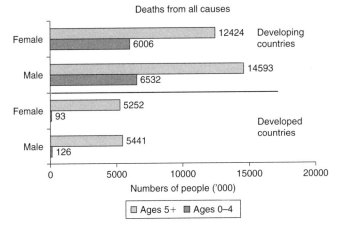

The following table shows the number of deaths caused by respiratory diseases in the world (in thousands) for the same time period as the graph above. Malignancy of trachea, bronchus and lung and COPD are smoking-related diseases.

Cause of death	Developing Countries				Developed Countries			
	Male		Female		Male		Female	
	Ages 0–4	Age 5+	Ages 0–4	Age 5+	Ages 0–4	Age 5+	Ages 0–4	Age 5+
Tuberculosis (TB)	43	1094	39	746	0	29	0	9
Lower respiratory tract (LRT) Infections	1328	688	1229	670	12	168	8	196
Upper respiratory tract (URT) Infections	14	7	13	6	0	1	0	2
Malignancy of Trachea, Bronchus and Lung	0	309	0	113	0	399	0	124
COPD	17	991	23	855	0	206	0	119
Asthma	1	57	1	49	0	13	0	16

23 What is the ratio of the sex difference in respiratory diseases in those aged up to 4 to those aged 5 and above in developing countries?

 A 0.03
 B 0.14
 C 0.44
 D 0.53
 E 7

24 For males over 5 years, what is the difference between developed countries and developing countries in the proportion of respiratory deaths to deaths from all causes? (Give your answer to two decimal places.)

25 Assuming that the data above is accurate which one of the following can we safely conclude to be true?

 A Compared to those aged 5 and above, there were much greater gender differences in the mortality pattern in those aged up to 4 in both the developed and developing world.
 B Whereas deaths as a result of lung cancer and COPD were similar to those caused by TB in developing countries they were more than 50 times that caused by TB in the developed world.
 C The pattern of deaths from asthma between sexes for ages up to 4 was significantly different for developing and developed world.
 D Compared to the developing world, smoking-related diseases have a greater significance in causing respiratory diseases than TB.

26 **Argument**
Illusions and magic tricks are entertaining spectacles but should not be viewed by anything other than sceptical eyes. The very word "trick" express the fact that the viewer is being duped, that the magician is playing an intellectual joke.

Statement
The words "magic" and "trick" are contradictory: while the former suggests something supernatural the latter suggests deception.

Which of the following best describes how the short statement relates to the argument?

 A Restates the main conclusion.
 B Presents a serious challenge.
 C Lends qualified support.
 D Paraphrases one of argument's main premises.

27 A circle can be divided into a maximum of four sections and seven sections using two straight lines and three straight lines respectively as shown in the diagram below. What is the maximum number of sections that can be obtained using four straight lines?

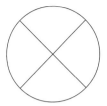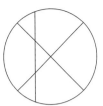

A 8
B 9
C 10
D 11
E 12

28 The pattern below is a representative sample of a design which is covering a large area on the ceiling of a building.

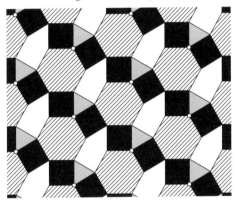

What ratio of individual tiles, shown below, makes up the design?

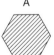

Questions 29 and 30 refer to the information below:

A sample of 100 individuals was classified into groups based on several criteria. Each of the graphs below compares the presence of two features among the group. Each quadrant represents the number of people who are positive or negative for one feature and positive or negative for the other.

For example, in Graph 1 the top left quadrant shows that there are 59 individuals who are male and not female, while the bottom half of Graph 2 shows that there are 89 people who do not have asthma and in Graph 3 the bottom right quadrant shows that there are 21 people who are female and do not have a squint.

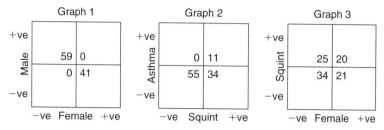

Graph 1   Graph 2   Graph 3

29 What fraction of the people who do not have a squint are male?

A 0.2
B 0.3
C 0.4
D 0.6
E 0.9

30 If the proportion of the sample population that are male, have a squint AND do not have asthma amounts to 22%, what percentage of females are asthmatic?

A 7.3%
B 10%
C 19.5%
D 27%
E 37%

31 A government proposal has recently been put forward which would extend the time allowed for detention of criminals without trial from the current 14 days to 90 days. This is a welcome development indeed as the rapid advancement of modern technology has been exploited by terrorist organisations, which are now able to sustain networks spread across the world using highly sophisticated computer technology, encryption of documents and mobile phone communication which are all difficult to decipher and collate.

Which of the following best summarises the conclusion of the above argument?

A Ninety days is not long enough to detain suspected terrorists because their networks may be spread over many countries.
B In the event of a major terrorist atrocity, the government would enforce martial law in order to protect its citizens.
C Terrorist organisations are centrally controlled and it is more difficult for law enforcement agencies to gather enough evidence to bring suspects to trial.

D Extra work has to be done to collate data from suspects which may be spread over a wide area or need decoding by specialists, which would take longer than previously.
E The time currently allowed for detention without trial is inadequate and therefore an extension is imperative.

32 In some countries there is a time bomb waiting to explode: a population time bomb. This cataclysm does not involve numbers reaching for the stars, but sex; sex ratios to be precise. In China and India, for example, which have for so long favoured males over their female siblings, there seems to be a skew emerging, which may have dangerous consequences. In some parts of these countries, there are two males born for every female. It may be that in a population composed of so many surplus men, the women are able to select their partners with more scrutiny than they may have done in a less biased gender divide. One can envisage a country full of single men with nothing to do. Examples from history have shown, that in other societies this has lead to civil unrest, violence and crime. The security implications are therefore too important to be ignored in two of the most populous countries on earth.

Even if the evidence is correct, which of the following show that the conclusion is unsafe?

(i) It may be the case that females have a pacifying influence on males.
(ii) It may be the case that in the past civil unrest, violence and crime were commonplace in all societies.
(iii) It may be the case that violent societies prefer male offspring.

A i only
B i and ii only
C ii and iii only
D i and iii only
E i, ii and iii

Questions 33 to 35 refer to the following information:

Wine is made by fermenting the juice of the grape of the vine *Vitis vinifera*. Although it has been made for over 7,000 years, it is the least consumed of the three types of alcoholic beverages, accounting for less than one seventh of the world's consumption of alcohol in the 1960s; since then world per capita consumption had nearly halved by the late 1990s.

There are many reasons for the variations in the consumption of alcoholic beverages. In the case of international variations, however, consumption patterns are often related to production, due, until recently, to the high cost of transporting beverages over long distances. This is true of wine; until the 1960s 90% of all wine output was consumed in the country where it was produced, although a greater proportion of the *value* of output was exported; the trade in wine between southern and northern Europe has existed for at least a millennium. There is a high correlation between the present production and consumption in spite of the increase in proportion of production exported, which nearly reached a quarter in the late 1990s. Another factor explaining the variation in alcohol consumption has been migration; in the case of wine specifically the migration of Europeans to non-producing areas.

Beer is the leading drink in northern Europe and North America. The advent of the railway and the motorway has reduced the cost of transport and conveying beer in bottles, cans and kegs rather than casks has reduced the rate of deterioration. Even so there is still a very high correlation between consumption per capita and output per capita at a national level.

Spirits are made by distilling fermented beverage and in contrast to wine, and beer made from barley malt, spirits can be made from a great variety of plants. Although Scotch whiskey and French brandy are exported all over the world, a surprisingly small proportion of world spirit production is exported. The location of production is not a powerful factor in explaining the variation of consumption as it is with beer or wine, and income per capita seems to have very little influence international variations.

Adapted from *Wine, Spirits and Beer* David Grigg.

33 If in the 40 years preceding the end of the last millennium, the world population increased by a factor of 6 and the combined global consumption of beer and spirits increased by a factor of 7, approximately what fraction of the total world consumption of alcohol did the consumption of spirits and beer account for in year 2000?

A 3/49
B 3/42
C 2/7
D 6/7
E 14/15

34 Which of the following can least reliably be inferred from the passage?

A French brandy and Scotch whiskey belong to the same family of alcoholic beverages.
B The world consumption of wines in 1960 was less than half the highest consumed of the main types of alcoholic beverage.
C In the 1950s the proportion of the value of produced wine that was exported exceeded 10%.
D There is still a correlation between the production of alcohol and the consumption of the same per capita on a national level.
E Beer is the highest produced alcoholic beverage in North America and northern Europe.

35 If alcoholic beverages were listed in order of worldwide consumption from highest to the lowest, which of the following are compatible with the given information?

A Beer, Wine, Spirits
B Spirits, Beer, Wine
C Beer, French Brandy, Wine, Scotch Whiskey
D Scotch Whiskey, Beer, French Brandy, Wine

END OF SECTION 1

SAMPLE PAPER B

SECTION 2B Scientific Knowledge and Application

Response Sheet

With questions like these fill in the appropriate bubble with your chosen answer e.g.

A B C D
○ ● ○ ○

With questions like these, write your answer clearly in the space provided with one letter or digit in each space. Use BLOCK CAPITALS

| 4 | 3 | . | 2 | 5 |

Name

Date Of Birth

1   A B C D
    ○ ○ ○ ○

2   A B C D E F
    ○ ○ ○ ○ ○ ○

3   A B C D
    ○ ○ ○ ○

4   i ☐ ii ☐

    iv ☐ v ☐

5   A B C D E F
    ○ ○ ○ ○ ○ ○

6   A B C D E
    ○ ○ ○ ○ ○

7   A B C D E
    ○ ○ ○ ○ ○

8   A B C D
    ○ ○ ○ ○

9   ☐☐☐☐☐☐ Ω

10 A B C D E
    ○ ○ ○ ○ ○

11 A B C D E
    ○ ○ ○ ○ ○

12 A B C D E
    ○ ○ ○ ○ ○

13 A B C D E
    ○ ○ ○ ○ ○

14 A B C D E
    ○ ○ ○ ○ ○

15 A B C D E F G
    ○ ○ ○ ○ ○ ○ ○

16 ☐☐ : ☐☐ : ☐☐ : ☐☐

17 ☐☐☐☐☐☐

18 A B C D E
    ○ ○ ○ ○ ○

19 A B C D E
    ○ ○ ○ ○ ○

20 A B C D E
    ○ ○ ○ ○ ○

21 p ☐☐ q ☐☐

22 A B C D E
    ○ ○ ○ ○ ○

23 A B C D E
    ○ ○ ○ ○ ○

24 ☐☐☐☐☐☐

25 A B C D E
    ○ ○ ○ ○ ○

26 A B C D E F G
    ○ ○ ○ ○ ○ ○ ○

27 A B C D E F G
    ○ ○ ○ ○ ○ ○ ○

Paper 2B   30 minutes

SECTION 2   Scientific Knowledge and Application

Instructions to Candidates

Please read this page carefully. Speed as well as accuracy is important in this section. ***Work quickly, or you may not finish the paper***. There are no penalties for incorrect responses, only points for correct answers, so you should attempt all 27 questions.

Unless otherwise stated, all questions are worth one mark.

Answer on the sheet provided. Many questions ask you to show your choice between options by shading a circle (or circles, if specified in the question).

If questions ask you to write in words or numbers be sure to write clearly in the spaces provided.

Choose the option which best answers the question asked. If you make a mistake, erase it thoroughly and try again.

Calculators are *not* permitted.

1 The diagram below shows a schematic representation of the menstrual cycle in humans.

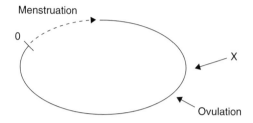

Which row in the following table depicts the hormonal balance at X?

	Oestrogen	Progesterone	LH	FSH
A	high	low	high	high
B	high	high	high	low
C	low	high	high	high
D	high	low	low	high

2 Which of the following are correct simplifications of the equation:

$$\frac{2}{x + 5} + \frac{x + 4}{4} = \frac{8}{x + 5}$$

A $x^2 + 9x - 4 = 0$
B $9(x + 4) = 4$
C $x^2 + 11x + 14 = 0$
D $30(x + 5) = -2$
E $(x + 7)(x + 4) = 14$
F $(x + 4)(x + 5) - 20 = 0$

3 Which two of the following are equivalent?

A (Force/Time) × Distance
B Force/Mass
C (Current)^2 × Resistance
D Energy/Charge

4 The results of an experiment to test the electrical conductivity of five substances are listed in the table below:

Substance	Conductivity	Reason
Copper sulphate crystals	Non-conductor	i
Iron nail	Conductor	ii
Sodium chloride solution	Conductor	iii
Sugar solution	Non-conductor	iv
Wax	Non-conductor	v

Choose the correct statement (**A** to **D**) from the list below to explain the results in the numbered spaces (**i** to **v**). Each statement may be used once, more than once or not at all.

A Because it contains ions that are free to move.
B Because it contains delocalised electrons which are free to move.
C Because it contains ions that are not free to move.
D Because it does not contain ions.

5 In a clinical trial to test the metabolism of a new drug – DX450 – 10 ml of the substance is injected into a vein in a subject's right arm. Which of the following is compatible with the movement of DX450 within the subject's circulatory system, assuming only one passage via the heart is permitted?

A Abdominal capillary bed → Abdominal venules → Right ventricle → Pulmonary vein → Pulmonary valve
B Aorta → Cerebral (brain) artery → Right atrium → Left atrium → Aortic valve
C Pulmonary artery → Left atrium → Right ventricle → Pulmonary vein → Left arm vein
D Right arm vein → Leg vein → Abdominal artery → Right ventricle → Aorta
E Right arm vein → Right hand vein → Pulmonary artery → Left atrium → Atrio-ventricular valve
F Right atrium → Pulmonary artery → Left ventricle → Aorta → Retinal (eye) venules

6 When $y = 0$, $x = 3$ or -3. What is the value of y when $x = 0$?

A -9
B -3
C 0
D 3
E 9

7 In a series of experiments, three gases are produced and collected in separate test tubes. The tubes have been labelled P, Q and R. It is known that the gases are oxygen, carbon dioxide and hydrogen but it is not known which gas occupies which test tube. Which single test out of the options listed below (**A** to **E**) can be used to distinguish these three gases apart?

A Expose each gas to a glowing splint and observe the results.
B Expose each gas to a lighted splint and observe the results.
C Bubble each gas through limewater and observe the results.
D Mix each gas with bromine water and observe the results.
E Expose each gas to moist blue litmus paper and observe the results.

8 Urine is collected from four subjects (**P** to **S**) over 6 hours under equivalent standard conditions. Subject **P** is a normal control.

	P	Q	R	S
Urine volume (ml)	500	40	1200	50
Concentration of sodium (standard units)	0	50	100	200
Concentration of urea (standard units)	100	50	20	200

Which part(s) of the renal system could be defective (i.e. performing less of their normal function) in subject **Q**?

A Glomerulus
B Proximal tubules
C Collecting duct
D Blood supply (Renal arteries)

9 The diagram below shows a device consisting of three transformers connected in series. The voltmeter is being used to measure the output voltage.

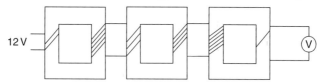

What is the resistance of the voltmeter, if it draws a current of 2 A from the device? Give your answer correct to 2 decimal places.

10 The following table shows typical properties of certain cell types. Which of the following options (**A** to **E**) is most likely to refer to **animal cells**?

	A	B	C	D	E
Possesses a cell wall	○	●	○	○	●
Possesses nucleic acids	●	●	●	●	●
Contains chloroplasts	○	●	●	○	○
Structurally composed of protein	●	●	●	●	●
Possesses vacuoles	●	●	○	○	●

Key
● Yes
○ No

11 Which one of the following is a means of heat transfer which does not require a substance to transfer heat?

A Sublimation
B Conduction
C Radiation
D Convection
E Refraction

12 The boxes below show functions for two separate variables, y and z.

$$y = (x + 4)(x + 3)$$

$$z = 2x + 14 + \frac{24}{x}$$

What function needs to be applied to y in order that $y = z$?

A $\frac{2}{x} y + 1$

B $\frac{2}{x} y$

C $2y$

D $y - 5x + 2 - x^2$

E $y - 5x + 2 + \frac{24}{x}$

13 Below is a wave of speed $16\,\text{m/s}$. This is the way the wave looks at time $t = 0\,\text{s}$:

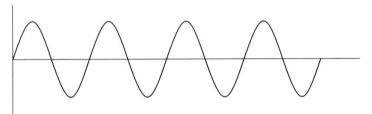

This is the way it looks after time $t = 4\,\text{s}$:

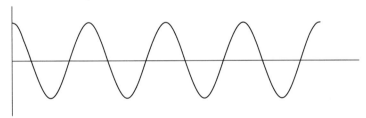

This is the way it looks after time $t = 8\,\text{s}$:

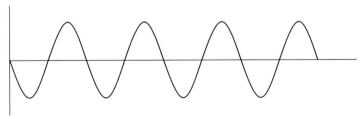

At which of the following times will it look exactly like it looked at time
t = 0 s?

A t = 40 s
B t = 56 s
C t = 72 s
D t = 144 s
E t = 178 s

14 After ingesting alcohol, detoxification in the liver occurs in several met-
abolic steps. These include the conversion of ethanol, C_2H_6O, to acetaldehyde, C_2H_4O (reaction 1), the conversion of acetaldehyde to acetate,
$C_2H_4O_2$ (reaction 2) and the conversion of acetate to acetyl CoA. The
acetyl CoA is then used in the citric acid cycle, and converted to CO_2.

Which of the following accurately represents the chemical changes
occurring in reactions 1 and 2?

	Reaction 1	Reaction 2
A	Oxidation	Reduction
B	Reduction	Oxidation
C	Dehydration	Reduction
D	Reduction	Reduction
E	Oxidation	Oxidation

15 If the "widget" (a new physical quantity) of the car below at any given
point is defined as the product of its acceleration at that point and the distance covered up to that point (from point 1), at which single point (**A** to
G) on the graph below does the car have the highest "widget" value?

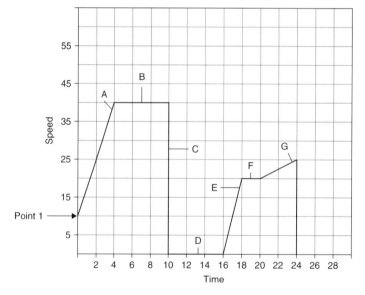

16 The four circuits shown below are each composed of two identical cells and two identical resistors arranged in different ways. What is the ratio of the **power** used in resistors $R_A:R_B:R_C:R_D$?

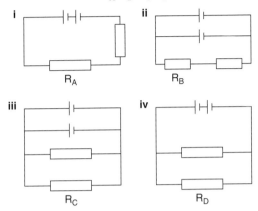

17 A microphone can be modelled as a sphere on top of a closed cone, as shown in figure 1 below. Using the values given in figure 2, calculate the surface area to volume ratio of the microphone model. Assume that the surface contact between cone and sphere is negligible. Express your answer accurate to 3 decimal places.

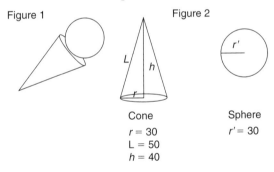

Figure 1   Figure 2

Cone
$r = 30$
$L = 50$
$h = 40$

Sphere
$r' = 30$

18 Zinc and sulphuric acid are reacted to produce hydrogen in the apparatus as shown in the diagram below.

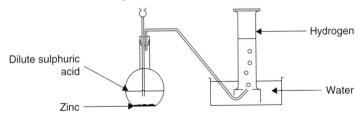

Dilute sulphuric acid

Zinc

Hydrogen

Water

Several experiments are performed under different conditions as shown in the table below. The only variables are temperature, form of zinc used, and dilutions of sulphuric acid (the total volume of $50\,cm^3$ is used made up of varying proportions of pure water and $2\,mol/dm^3$ sulphuric acid). A fixed time period is used to collect the gas and none of the experiments have enough time to reach completion.

	Acid volume	Water volume	Temperature/°C	Zinc form
i	$50\,cm^3$	$0\,cm^3$	50	Chips
ii	$20\,cm^3$	$30\,cm^3$	50	Chips
iii	$30\,cm^3$	$20\,cm^3$	10	Chips
iv	$20\,cm^3$	$30\,cm^3$	50	Powder
v	$50\,cm^3$	$0\,cm^3$	100	Chips

The experiments are ranked according to the volume of hydrogen produced. Which of the following is compatible with the data for volume of hydrogen gas produced (ordered from highest volume to lowest volume of gas collected)?

A i, ii, iv, v
B ii, iii, i
C iii, ii, iv, v
D iv, iii, ii, v
E v, i, ii

19 Using a Geiger counter, background radiation is defined as <0.05 arbitrary units. If a certain radioactive substance has a half life of 16 years and the starting level of radioactivity is 250 arbitrary units, how many years before the radiation emitted from the substance is indistinguishable from the background radiation?

A 160
B 168
C 184
D 194
E 224

20 The diagram shows a triangle with its base on the diameter of a circle.

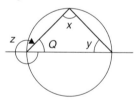

Which of the following statements are true?

A $\sin y = \cos Q$
B $\sin Q = \sin(180+Q)$
C $\cos Q = \cos z$
D $\cos Q = \cos(x+y)$
E $\tan y = \tan z$

21 The regular solid box shown below exerts a pressure of 5.5 Pa on the ground. Assuming acceleration of free fall is 10 m/s², what is the density of the object? Convert your answer to the form, $p \times 10^q$, giving values for p and q.

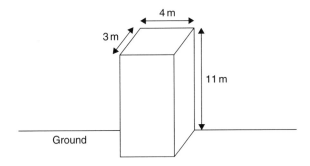

22 A biochemical reaction is being investigated to determine the rates of reaction under different conditions. Two sets of reactions are carried out at pH 4 and at pH 8. In each set the reactants are either mixed with solution X, containing only enzyme A, or solution Y, containing a combination of enzymes A, B and C. The graphs below summarise the results of the reactions.

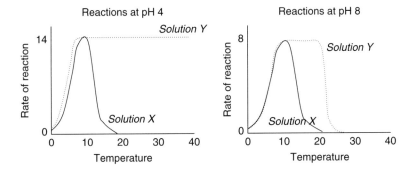

Based on the information shown, which of the following statements could be true?

A Enzymes B and C do not denature, whilst enzyme A does.

B All three enzymes are active at pH 4 whilst only two are active at pH 8.

C Enzyme B works better than enzyme A at low pH.

D At 50°C solution X will probably be active.

E The enzymes would work just as well with different substrates.

23 Which of the following participants at a weightlifting competition is the most powerful? (Assume $g = 10\,\text{m/s}^2$)

	A	B	C	D	E
Weight rating of each dumbbell (kg)	30	25	35	40	30
Number of dumbbells lifted	4	6	4	4	6
Weight of participant (kg)	120	90	85	150	105
Distance dumbbells lifted (m)	2	1.5	1	2.2	1.4
Time taken to lift dumbbells (min)	20	25	15	30	20

24 The graph below shows the velocity of a missile. What is the average acceleration of the missile in miles/minute² over the first 4 minutes? Give your answer correct to 2 decimal places.

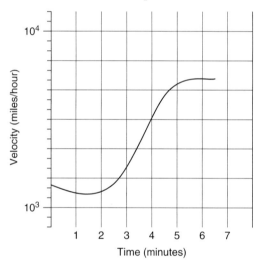

25 The enzyme carbonic anhydrase (C.A.) catalyses the forward reaction:

$$CO_2 + H_2O \rightarrow H^+ + HCO_3^-$$

The following diagram shows the reversible reaction occurring in the distal convoluted tubule cells of the kidney, catalysed by carbonic anhydrase:

Which of the following would cause the intracellular concentration of HCO_3^- to increase?

A A decrease in intracellular pH from 7.3 to 7.2.
B An increase in removal of H^+ from the cell?
C A drug which inhibits the enzyme C.A.
D An increase in CO_2 production.
E An increase in temperature from 37°C to 74°C.

26 Which of the following options **A** to **G** is the most accurate description of the eye of a short-sighted person?

	Strength of lens	Eye length	Light rays focussed relative to retina	Corrective lens
A	Too strong	Too short	In front	Diverging
B	Too weak	Too short	Behind	Converging
C	Too strong	Too long	In front	Concave
D	Too strong	Too short	Behind	Convex
E	Normal	Too long	In front	Concave
F	Too weak	Too long	Behind	Biconcave
G	Too weak	Too long	In front	Diverging

27 The diagram below shows the fractional distillation of crude oil (X) which is pumped in at the bottom of the tower.

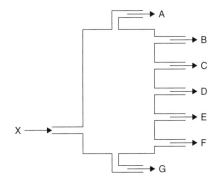

Which statements about the fractional distillation of crude oil are true?

(i) Shorter molecules condense at lower temperatures.
(ii) Molecules of D are less flammable than molecules of C.
(iii) The boiling point of molecules of F is higher than molecules of A.

A i only
B ii and iii only
C i and iii only
D i and ii only
E i, ii and iii

END OF SECTION 2

Paper 3B   30 minutes

SECTION 3   Writing Task

Instructions to Candidates

This question paper contains a choice of three tasks, of which you must answer only **one**. It also provides space in which you may make any preliminary notes you wish, but your answer must be written on a single page of an A4 sheet.

The tasks each provide an opportunity for you to show how well you can:

● select, develop and organise ideas and
● communicate them effectively in writing.

Before you begin writing, think carefully about what you need to say and the ways in which the organisation and layout of your response might help convey your message, diagrams, etc. may be used if they enhance communication.

Take care to show how well you can write and be concise, clear and accurate.

Dictionaries may NOT be used.

Remember that when you are told that you may begin you will have only 30 minutes to choose and complete your task, and that your complete response must be contained on a single side of an A4 sheet. The disciplines involved in this are regarded as key features of the task.

YOU MUST ANSWER ONLY <u>ONE</u> OF THE FOLLOWING QUESTIONS

1 The phenomenal development of the technology of information has changed the nature of education in modern society; inspiration is the last vestigial role of the teacher.

Write a unified essay in which you address the following:

What do you think this statement means and why do you think the author holds this viewpoint? Advance an argument against this viewpoint, i.e. inspiration is not the last vestigial role of the teacher.

2 **History is a harsh tutor as her instruction cannot be understood till the lesson is finished.**

Write a unified essay in which you address the following:

What do you understand by this statement? What is the distinction between "instruction" and "lesson" as used in this statement? Advance a counter-argument, i.e. that her instruction can be understood before the lesson is finished.

3. **Decision making in society is the privilege of the few; it should be the prerogative of the many.**

Write a unified essay in which you address the following:

What do you think this statement means? What do you understand by "decision making" as used in this statement? Advance a counter-argument, i.e. that decision making should be the privilege of the few.

END OF SECTION 3
END OF PAPER 2

CHAPTER 8
UKCAT practice papers

PRACTICE QUESTIONS

SAMPLE PAPER 1

Verbal Reasoning Instructions

In this section of the exam, you will be presented passages to read. For each passage, there will be four statements relating to the text. Your task is to decide whether the statements follow logically from the information in the passage. For each statement, there are three answer options.

Option A – True: This means that, on the basis of the information in the passage, the statement is true or logically follows from the passage.

Option B – False: This means that, on the basis of the information in the passage, the statement is false.

Option C – Can't tell: This means that you cannot tell from the information in the passage whether the statement is true or false.

When deciding on whether a statement is True (A), False (B) or Can't tell (C), it is important to base your answer only on information in the passage and not on any other knowledge you may have. This information may be found within the question.

You will have 21 minutes to answer 44 questions. It is in your best interest to answer all items as there is no penalty for guessing. All unanswered items will be scored as incorrect.

Item 1

The development of toothpaste began as long ago as 500 BC in China and India. It was known even back then, in China, that cleaning the teeth could alleviate toothache. Crushed bone, crushed egg and oyster shells, were some of the things used to clean debris from teeth. Tooth powders were the next step in teeth hygiene, consisting of powdered charcoal, powdered bark and some flavouring agents. This would be applied to teeth using a simple stick. Toothpowder or dentifrice was first available in Britain in the late 18th century; it usually came in a ceramic pot and was available either as a powder or paste. The rich applied it with brushes and the poor with their fingers.

Modern toothpastes were developed in the 1800s. A dentist called Peabody was the first to add soap to toothpaste in 1824. Chalk was first added to toothpaste by John Harris in the 1850s. In 1873, toothpaste was first mass produced into nice smelling toothpaste in a jar.

1 Dentifrice was first available in Britain in the 1800s.
2 The development of toothpaste predated the development of toothbrushes.
3 By the introduction of toothpowder in Britain, only the rich could afford toothbrushes.
4 Dentifrice came before crushed bone.

Item 2

The Haber Process (or Haber-Bosch Process) is the chemical reaction between nitrogen and hydrogen to produce ammonia. The reaction is reversible, which means that although ammonia is formed in the "forward" reaction, it can just as readily "unreact", re-forming nitrogen and hydrogen, in the "reverse" reaction. The direction of the reaction depends on external conditions such as temperature and pressure.

Usually the reaction is carried out at between 450°C and 500°C and at pressures of 250 times atmospheric. An iron catalyst is used to increase the rate of ammonia production. Although a pressure of greater than 250 times atmospheric would result in more ammonia production, very high pressures are not economically beneficial. This is because the energy required to build a plant to withstand high pressures and to maintain high pressures would not outweigh the economic gains made from the increased production of ammonia.

Ammonia is vital for agriculture since it is used to make fertilisers. Our demand for fertilisers is so great that in 2002, 1% of the total world energy consumption was consumed in the Haber process.

1 The end product of the Haber process is fertiliser.
2 The iron catalyst increases the quantity of ammonia produced.
3 A reaction occurring at a pressure of 500 times atmospheric would be economically unviable.
4 Since 2002 world demand for fertilisers has increased.

Item 3

The skin is composed of several layers one of which is eponymously entitled the Malpighian layer after Italian anatomist Marcello Malpighi (1628–1694). While studying the skin, Malpighi also described the patterns on the finger pulps which were to be termed fingerprints by others in the late 19th century.

The characteristics of fingerprints are now routinely used to detect crime by matching suspects to the scene of a crime or to a murder weapon. Standard patterns such as loops and whorls as well as composite patterns have necessitated various classification systems to be developed. This ensures all prints can be categorised and hence identified with confidence between specimens.

1 Marcello Malpighi discovered fingerprints in all but name in Italy in the 17th century.
2 Fingerprints are a routine method of detecting crime in modern usage.
3 Loops, whorls and other composite patterns are standardised to ensure a classification system can be developed.
4 If the fingerprint patterns on a murder weapon match the fingerprint patterns of a suspect then that suspect is guilty of committing a crime.

Item 4

One reason which is sometimes used against the possibility of time travel and expanded upon by Steven Hawking is that if time travel were possible then where are all the time travel tourists? A similar argument is made to disprove the existence of intelligent life elsewhere in the universe: if there was intelligent life other than on this planet, Earth would be surrounded by aliens.

There are many reasons that could be used to explain why time travel is possible and yet there are apparently no time travellers amongst us. For example, it may be that time travel is only possible into the future and not into the past. Alternatively, the laws of time travel may be such that one can only travel back in time to the point at which one invented a time machine and no further. Since no time machine yet exists, there will be no time travel tourists.

1 Time travel, argues Steven Hawking, is impossible.
2 Intelligent life must not exist elsewhere in the universe if aliens have not visited Earth in great numbers.
3 Time travel is governed by laws which state that one can only move forward in time.
4 If a time machine had been invented in the future we would have heard about it by now.

Item 5

Killing another person is often seen as inexcusable and wrong. However, many countries still enforce the death penalty. Although it seems common-sense for society to have some restriction on killing other people, the rules vary greatly between cultures and across the ages. Killing a human is seen as worse than killing an animal or plant. However in some cases merely belonging to the species *Homo sapiens* does not necessarily imbue a person's life with intrinsic value. For example, the Greeks and Romans would routinely sacrifice slaves, deformed newborns or so-called "barbarians" guided by dogma which changed from time to time. The only tempering of this view was brought about by religious concepts of immortal souls and that to kill a person usurps the position of God to decide when we live and die.

1   Countries which still support the death penalty are acting against common-sense.

2   Killing animals is more acceptable than killing humans because animals do not feel pain.

3   The ancient Greeks and Romans were not Christian because they routinely killed humans.

4   A "barbarian" although belonging to the species *Homo sapiens* was not considered as having human value.

Item 6

Consumers becoming more environmentally friendly have driven a move towards "greener" chemicals by manufacturers and retailers. Customers that demand a company with an environmental conscience will be listened to if it means larger profits for the businesses concerned.

   Environmental groups like Greenpeace advise companies about reducing certain harmful chemicals from the product repertoire. Natural chemicals like citric acid are less complex than synthetic chemicals, more easily broken down and less polluting. Such biodegradable ingredients in products ranging from toilet cleaner to kitchen disinfectant are proving to be just as effective and certainly more popular.

1   Concern for the environment by large companies is fuelling consumer opinion to purchase new "greener" products.

2   If customers do not demand a company to have scruples concerning the environment, businesses will not change their practices.

3   Citric acid is less polluting than other chemicals because it is less complex.

4   New "green" products have to be biodegradable in order to be popular.

Item 7

Imports of olive oil to the US in the early eighties were approximately 10 million gallons. A decade and a half later the figure was five times that amount. Although olive cultivation originated in Syria, the major producers are now Spain, Italy and Greece. Indeed, the Mediterranean rim accounts for 99% of all olive oil. Two tons of olives picked from the olive trees of the Andalusian hills of Spain for example give about a hundred gallons of oil. The freshly picked olives are crushed whole (including the pit). The solid is separated from the liquid and then the water is separated from the oil. This is then bottled for consumption.

A secondary benefit to Italians or Spaniards, to whom olive oil is regarded as the essence of a meal, is the healthy properties it is perceived to have. The high concentration of monounsaturated fat (the healthy sort) and antioxidants (such as vitamin E) and the lack of cholesterol may be the reason for the lowest rate of heart disease in Mediterranean people compared to other Western nations.

1 Olive oil imports to the US peaked in the early eighties.
2 At least half of the olive oil produced comes from the Andalusian hills.
3 By 1995 over 100,000 tons of olives were picked from olive trees just to satisfy the American market for olive oil.
4 The most important reason Italians and Spaniards consume olive oil is to reduce their risk of heart disease.

Item 8

The term "elitist" and the concept of elitism has colloquially become a term of abuse. Popularly many people believe that elitism is the same as belonging to a hereditary class system and having an elevated position as a consequence of birthright. Strictly speaking however elitism is the belief that a society should contain groups of people pre-eminent in any given field. Thus specialisation in medicine, politics the arts and other areas leads to an elite cadre in these areas. Unless those members of the hereditary class system have any particular talent they do not, technically, belong to an elite. Indeed, the existence of an elite should make it possible for any person of any class to reach any position in society if they have the talent. Hence, if certain conditions exist such as the ability to nurture talent and the presence of social mobility then the natural variation among human talents which occur should inevitably lead to elitism.

1 Elitism is misunderstood by the public as a whole.
2 The concept of elitism is to produce a subgroup of the population who excel in a particular field.
3 Those who fear the true meaning of elitism are the people considered elite by the misinformed public.
4 Being called "elitist" could be seen as derogatory.

Item 9

In ancient Greece many people conspicuous by their valour or conquests were honoured by being crowned with a wreath of laurel or bay leaves. This plant was sacred to the god Apollo. In ancient mythology, Apollo was the Greek and Roman god of the sun as well as being the god most closely associated with the arts. In the 15th century a new term was coined: "laureate" which was attributed to "a person worthy of receiving laurels" which was conferred on various poets.

   This title, Poet Laureate, still exists today, but the modern status of the title was only acquired in the late 17th century. At this time the Poet Laureate was granted a stipend as a member of the royal household and it was within his bailiwick to write verses celebrating noteworthy occasions. The Romantic poet William Wordsworth was the first Poet Laureate to accept his appointment on the condition that he was not obliged to compose poetry specifically for special occasions, but others have continued the practice.

1 Apollo was the Roman sun god with some association with the art of poetry.
2 The ancient Greeks honoured all those who were strong and brave with laurel wreaths.
3 All Poet Laureates had the responsibility of creating poems commemorating royal events.
4 Wordsworth made sure he never composed poetry specifically for special occasions.

Item 10

The price of oil changes depending on the supply of and demand for petroleum which themselves are affected by many factors. Oil is bought and sold on international commodity markets. If people want more oil than producers can supply, prices go up (and vice versa) because petrol comes from oil and the prices people pay at the pump generally reflects the price of oil in the commodity markets.

   Most oil production is controlled by OPEC which can modulate the supply of oil to keep prices relatively stable. Sometimes demand rises so much or so quickly that organised attempts at tweaking supply is ineffective in stopping prices rising. On the other hand uncontrollable events such as natural disasters mean supply falls too drastically for anything to be done about it.

1 When the supply of oil increases the price of oil drops.
2 OPEC is the main factor controlling the price of oil on the international market.
3 The price of oil is kept relatively stable.
4 It is not always possible to control the price of oil.

Item 11

Cinnamon bark is widely used as a spice. Strictly speaking though, only Sri Lankan cinnamon bark is deserving of the name. There are related species of cinnamon known as cassia which is sometimes sold labelled as cinnamon. It is easy to distinguish cinnamon from cassia when the whole bark is examined. However, since much of the cinnamon sold is already processed as a ground spice it is more difficult to tell powered cinnamon from powdered cassia.

Cinnamon sticks can easily be ground into a powder using a spice grinder. If the same is attempted with cassia the spice grinder is likely to be damaged since cassia sticks are harder and thicker. If you suspect that your powdered cinnamon is actually powdered cassia, the iodine test (for starch) can be performed. This involves adding orange iodine to the powder in question. If it turns blue–black, this indicates cassia: with pure cinnamon the iodine remains orange.

1 Most of the spice sold with the cinnamon label is actually cassia.
2 Cassia and cinnamon are not indistinguishable.
3 Cassia sticks are so hard that they can damage spice grinders.
4 Cinnamon does not contain any starch.

END OF VERBAL REASONING SECTION

Quantitative Reasoning Instructions

In this section of the exam, you will be presented with charts and graphs that contain data. This information may be found within the question. For each chart or graph there will be four items, each with five answer options. Your task is to choose the best option.

You will have 21 minutes to answer 40 questions. It is in your best interest to answer all items as there is no penalty for guessing. All unanswered items will be scored as incorrect.

Calculators are permitted.

Item 1

The chart shows the average sale value (in thousands of pounds) for houses sold in two towns, Whittlesford and New Port between the months of January and June.

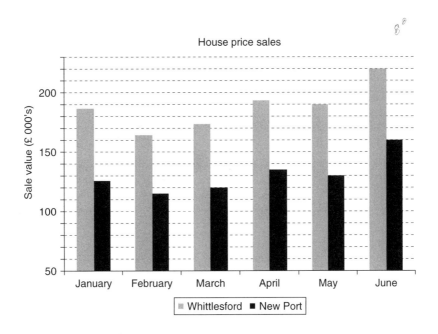

1 During which month was the average house sale price highest in Whittlesford?

   A January
   B March
   C April
   D May
   E June

2 Between which of the two months below was there the greatest absolute change in average sale price in New Port?

   A January–February
   B February–March
   C March–April
   D April–May
   E May–June

3 What is the percentage difference in average house price between the two towns at the beginning of the year (expressed in terms of the New Port price)?

A 20%
B 30%
C 40%
D 50%
E 60%

4 What is the average change in sale price over the 6 months for both towns?

A £20,000
B £25,000
C £30,000
D £35,000
E £40,000

Item 2

The table below shows electricity consumption for households in the state of Oberfranken over a 5-year period.

Electricity consumption per household (1,000 MW)		
	mean	range
1994	400	398–402
1995	385	365–405
1996	484	452–491
1997	542	520–568
1998	650	600–684

1 What was the average total consumption per household in MW over the 5 years?

A 2,461,000
B 2,486,000
C 2,435,000
D 2,412,000
E Can't tell

2 During which year did household consumption vary the most?

A 1995
B 1996
C 1997
D 1998
E Can't tell

3 Between which 2 years was there the greatest percentage increase in total consumption?

 A 1994–1995
 B 1995–1996
 C 1996–1997
 D 1997–1998
 E Can't tell

4 If mean household consumption followed the same overall trend in absolute terms, what would the predicted mean household consumption be in 2003?

 A 800
 B 950
 C 1,150
 D 1,420
 E 1,500

Item 3

The table shows a record of time (in hours) and cost (in £) for various jobs carried out by a repair-man, including estimates for each job made before undertaking them.

Job	Estimated		Actual	
	Time (hours)	Cost (£)	Time (hours)	Cost (£)
Wardrobe	16	350	32	120
Garage door	15	300	20	200
Leaking tap	0.5	5	0.25	2
Radiator	3	25	2	15
TV aerial	2	55	2.5	50
Insulation	10	200	8	150

1 What was the total time taken to complete all the jobs?

 A 45 hours 45 minutes
 B 46 hours 30 minutes
 C 55 hours 30 minutes
 D 62 hours 45 minutes
 E 64 hours 45 minutes

2 Which job was the most delayed?

 A Wardrobe
 B Garage door
 C Leaking tap
 D TV aerial
 E Insulation

3 What was the overall income per hour made by the repair-man in £?

  A 8.30
  B 8.50
  C 9.00
  D 9.20
  E 9.50

4 What was the difference between estimated and actual total cost per hour in £?

  A 6.15
  B 8.55
  C 8.62
  D 11.80
  E 21.80

Item 4

The following information shows the fees charged (in £'s) by a company for the sale of a property.

Item	Fee (£)
Estate agency	1% sale price
Solicitors	900.00
Search fees	250.00
Land registry	150.00
Mortgage assignment	100.00
Stamp duty	1% sale price
Valuation fee	350.00

1 What is the cost of the estate agent for a house sold at £167,000?

  A £167
  B £1,670
  C £16,700
  D £167,000
  E None of the above

2 What would be the most expensive item for a property worth £50,000?

  A Estate agent
  B Land registry
  C Solicitor
  D Stamp duty
  E Valuation

3 What would the total bill of fees come to, for a house worth £100,000?

    A £1,750
    B £2,000
    C £3,750
    D £4,500
    E £21,750

4 What is the percentage difference in stamp duty if a house's sale price rises from £100,000 to £120,000?

    A 10%
    B 20%
    C 30%
    D 40%
    E 50%

Item 5

The chart shows the dimensions of various rectangular boxes of equal height, with the number alongside each marker displaying the weight in kilograms.

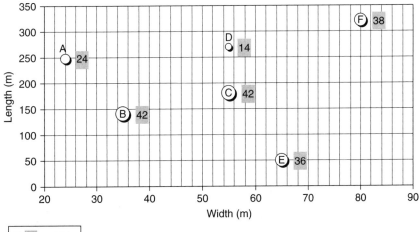

1 What are the dimensions of the heaviest box?

    A 35 m × 140 m × 55 m
    B 55 m × 180 m × 35 m
    C 80 m × 320 m × 55 m
    D 55 m × 270 m × 80
    E Can't tell

2 What is the average length of the boxes in metres?

 A 165
 B 182
 C 201
 D 218
 E 236

3 Which one of the following statements is true?

 A Box B could fit into Box A
 B Box C could fit into Box E
 C Box E could fit into Box C
 D Box B could fit into Box D
 E Box F could fit into Box D

4 Which box has the lowest density (mass for a given volume)?

 A Box A
 B Box B
 C Box C
 D Box D
 E Box E

Item 6

The table summarises viewing-figures for all BBC television channels.

	Channel	Average daily reach		Weekly reach		Average weekly viewing
		000s	%	000s	%	Hours:Minutes per person
Terrestrial	BBC 1	22,564	50.5	38,125	85.3	06:50
	BBC 2	12,184	27.3	29,847	66.8	02:20
Non-terrestrial	BBC 3	2,737	6.1	12,124	27.1	00:18
	BBC 4	852	1.9	4,359	9.8	00:05
	BBC News 24	2,313	5.2	7,888	17.6	00:14
	CBBC	855	1.9	3,219	7.2	00:08
	CBEEBIES	1,206	2.7	4,059	9.1	00:16
	Total terrestrial	28,455	63.7	40,175	89.9	17:26
	Total non-terrestrial	24,681	55.2	37,660	84.3	12:53

1 What is the difference between average weekly viewing per person for terrestrial BBC channels and non-terrestrial BBC channels?

 A 273
 B 305
 C 358
 D 405
 E 481

2 What proportion of total non-terrestrial TV viewing do the BBC channels account for?

    A 21%

    B 32%

    C 58%

    D 84%

    E Can't tell

3 What proportion of the day does an average person spend watching television?

    A 18%

    B 73%

    C 54%

    D >99% (virtually all day)

    E Can't tell

4 Of a group of 45 people who watch BBC 1 at least once during the week, how many of them on average would you expect to watch this channel on any given day?

    A 18

    B 21

    C 23

    D 26

    E Can't tell

Item 7

The table below shows mean times taken to travel between 3 hubs (A, B and C) by different airlines. Each journey is associated with a "delay" shown in brackets.

	Mean travel time (mean delay) in minutes			
Airline	A → B	A → C	B → C	B → A
Aerotravel	0:55 (0:30)	1:48 (0:32)	4:30 (0:47)	0:55 (0:50)
Akon	1:05 (0:34)	1:52 (0:35)	4:25 (0:52)	1:05 (0:48)
Celeriter	0:45 (0:30)	1:42 (0:28)	4:25 (0:55)	0:45 (0:52)
Douglas airlines	0:50 (0:28)	1:48 (0:29)	4:18 (0:46)	0:50 (0:51)
Jet air	1:02 (0:33)	1:51 (0:35)	4:38 (0:50)	1:02 (0:47)

1 Which airline, on average is associated with the greatest delay?

    A Aerotravel

    B Akon

    C Celeriter

    D Douglas Airlines

    E Jet Air

2 Which hub, on average is associated with the smallest delay?

 A Hub A
 B Hub B
 C Hub C
 D All hubs are associated with approximately equal delay
 E Can't tell

3 If I want to arrive at A by 09:20 a.m., which is the last plane I can catch from B without fear of being late?

 A Aerotravel service departing at 08:00
 B Akon service departing at 08:10
 C Celeriter service departing at 07:40
 D Celeriter service departing at 08:30
 E Jet Air service departing at 06:47

4 How many return journeys on average can I safely make from B to A with Jet airways in the same time it takes me to travel once from B to C using the same company?

 A 1
 B 2
 C 3
 D 4
 E Can't tell

Item 8

The chart below shows the relative contributions to GDP (gross domestic product) of various industries in the year 1998.

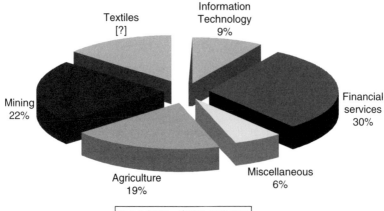

1   What is the GDP attributable to Textiles?

    A $15,000
    B $18,000
    C $20,000
    D Can't tell
    E None of the above

2   What is the greatest difference in GDP contribution between industries?

    A $380,000
    B $3,807,000
    C $3,960,000
    D $27,090,000
    E $30,960,000

3   If, the following year, total GDP falls by 12% and the relative contribution of Financial Services increases by 10% compared to its current contribution, what would be the approximate contribution of Financial Services in 1999?

    A 35 million
    B 37 million
    C 40 million
    D 42 million
    E 45 million

4   If over the next 5 years the proportion of Agriculture:Mining is projected to decrease by a proportion of 25%, whilst the contribution of Mining is projected to increase by a proportion of 50% of its current contribution, what would be the relative contribution of Agriculture in 5 years time?

    A 20%
    B 21%
    C 22%
    D 24%
    E 28%

Item 9

The table shows the base price and additional costs for 5 car models sold at Jimmy's car dealership. All values shown are in £.

Car model	Base cost	Optional extras						
		Leather seats	Air-conditioning or sunroof	Heated or electric seats	[combination supplement]	Metallic paint	Alloy wheels
ALFA	19,998.00	1,230.00	558.00	n/a	–	453.00	865.00
ESCORT	25,748.00	895.00	672.00	987.00	234.00	324.00	453.00
ORION	28,746.00	free	557.00	n/a	–	476.00	1,253.00
THRIFT	15,473.00	n/a	328.00	578.00	328.00	454.00	876.00
DOSKER	45,673.00	1,099.00	456.00	767.00	343.00	531.00	479.00

n/a: not available; "free": option included free of charge; the combination supplement is paid in addition if **both** heated and electric seats are required.

1 Which car is associated with the most expensive combination of optional extras? (Ignoring the combination supplement)

   A Alfa
   B Escort
   C Orion
   D Thrift
   E Dosker

2 A customer wants a car with leather seats, air-conditioning and heated and electric seats. He decides to buy the Escort. How much dearer would an Orion with the same specifications have been?

   A £378
   B £485
   C £870
   D £1,101
   E Can't tell

3 A car without alloy wheels depreciates at a rate of 10% a year and one with alloy wheels depreciates at a rate of 5% per year. What will be my total savings or losses over 3 years if I buy a **Basic** Orion with alloy wheels instead of one without alloy wheels? [Assuming there is no inflation]

   A £1,253 loss
   B £3,850 loss
   C £2,550 saving
   D £3,512 saving
   E £4,765 saving

4 Any car can be bought on a scheme of hire-purchase, whereby the total amount due is paid in monthly instalments over a 5-year period. Paying by this method also incurs an interest of 10%. If I buy an Alfa by hire-purchase, what would be the difference to my monthly premiums caused by adding all the available extras as opposed to getting the basic package?

A £52
B £57
C £65
D £70
E £77

Item 10

Cells grown in culture are tested for three antigens, Asp30, GQ3d and PAMP50. Presence of the antigen is marked "positive", absence of the antigen makes the cell "negative" for that antigen.

The following charts show the number of cells testing positive and negative for each antigen.

	PAMP50 positive	PAMP50 negative
Asp30 positive	19	100
Asp30 negative	81	0
GQ3d positive	45	24
GQ3d negative	55	76

1 How many cells were tested in total?

A 100
B 200
C 300
D 400
E Can't tell

2 What percentage of cells have only the GQ3d antigen?

A 0%
B 12%
C 24%
D 38.5%
E Can't tell

3 If in a separate group of PAMP50-positive cells, there are 20% fewer cells positive for Asp30 and 10% more cells positive for GQ3d, what is the ratio of Asp30 positive to GQ3d-positive cells in that group?

A 3:10
B 3:5
C 2:5
D 12:7
E 4:3

4 The total cost of producing a cell containing 2 antigens and 3 antigens are 2.5 times and 3.5 times respectively greater than the cost of producing a cell with a single antigen (which is $14). If all 19 Asp30-positive, PAMP50-positive cells are GQ3d positive, what is the total cost of producing the PAMP50-positive cell line?

A $2,611
B $4,562
C $5,383
D $6,447
E Can't tell

END OF QUANTITATIVE REASONING SECTION

Abstract Reasoning Instructions

In this section of the exam, you will be presented with two sets of shapes labelled "Set A" and "Set B". All the shapes in Set A are similar in some way, as are the shapes in Set B. Set A and Set B are not related to each other.

You have to work out in what way the shapes in Set A are similar to one another, and in what way the shapes in Set B are similar to each other. For the two sets of shapes, you will be shown five test shapes. Your task is to determine whether each test shape belongs to Set A (choose option A), Set B (choose option B), or neither set (choose option C).

You will have 15 minutes to answer 65 questions.

Item 1

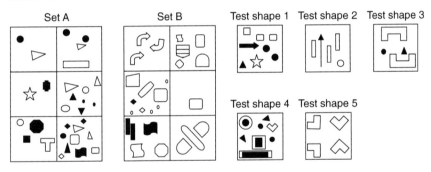

Item 2

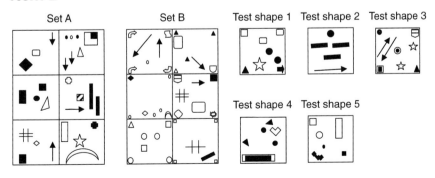

Item 3

Set A	Set B
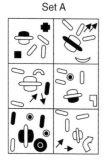	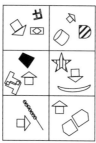

Test shape 1 Test shape 2 Test shape 3

Test shape 4 Test shape 5

Item 4

Set A	Set B
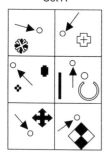	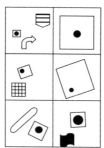

Test shape 1 Test shape 2 Test shape 3

Test shape 4 Test shape 5

Item 5

Set A	Set B
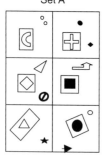	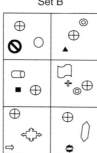

Test shape 1 Test shape 2 Test shape 3

Test shape 4 Test shape 5

Item 6

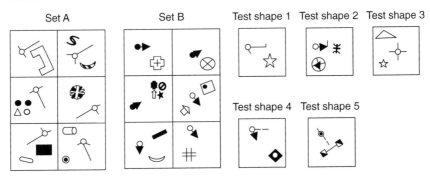

Set A   Set B   Test shape 1   Test shape 2   Test shape 3

Test shape 4   Test shape 5

Item 7

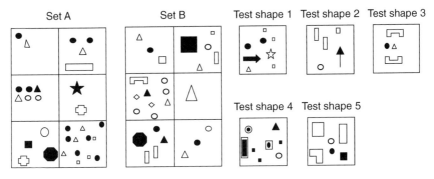

Set A   Set B   Test shape 1   Test shape 2   Test shape 3

Test shape 4   Test shape 5

Item 8

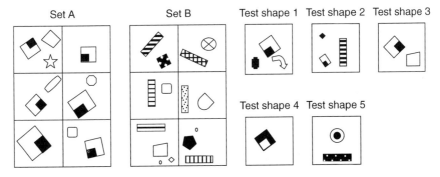

Set A   Set B   Test shape 1   Test shape 2   Test shape 3

Test shape 4   Test shape 5

Item 9

Set A	Set B	Test shape 1　Test shape 2　Test shape 3

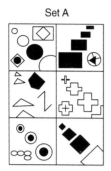
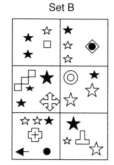
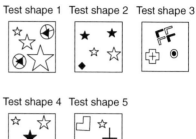

Test shape 4　Test shape 5

Item 10

Set A　　　　Set B　　Test shape 1　Test shape 2　Test shape 3

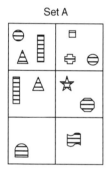
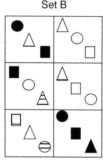
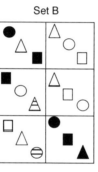
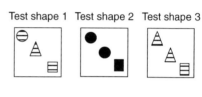

Test shape 4　Test shape 5

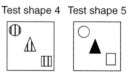

Item 11

Set A　　　　Set B　　Test shape 1　Test shape 2　Test shape 3

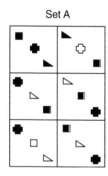
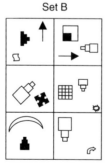
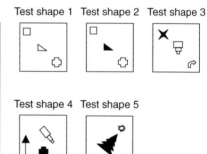

Test shape 4　Test shape 5

Item 12

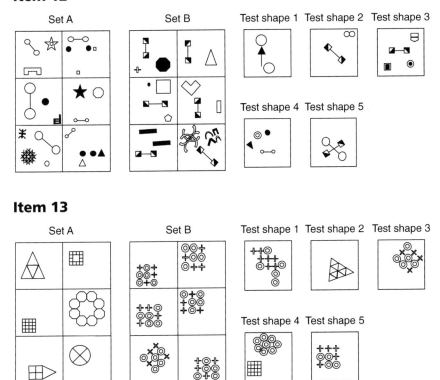

Item 13

END OF ABSTRACT REASONING SECTION

Decision Analysis Instructions

In this section of the exam, you will be presented with information relating to various problems. You will be asked to respond to a number of items relating to the information.

Your task is to choose the best option for each item.

For some of the questions you will have to select just one of the responses. For other questions you have to select more than one response.

You will have 29 minutes to answer 26 questions. It is in your best interest to answer all items as there is no penalty for guessing. All unanswered items will be scored as incorrect.

Table of codes

General rules	Basic codes
A = right	1 = transport
B = join	2 = man
C = plus	3 = land
D = slow	4 = down
E = total	5 = smoke
F = specific	6 = do
G = opposite	7 = train
	8 = post
	9 = close
	10 = joke
	11 = stay
	12 = strike
	13 = see
	14 = hear

1 What is the best interpretation of the following coded message: A2, 13, 4, E5

   A The smoke in the house was all around the man.
   B The good man could see down through all the smoke.
   C The man's visibility was down to a low level because of the smoke.
   D The man was overcome by all of the smoke.
   E The man looked right down and saw all the smoke.

2 What is the best interpretation of the following coded message: G(11), GA, 4CC, 3

   A Stay here deep in the field.
   B Don't stay here, go all the way down there.
   C Don't go the wrong way into the big building.
   D Turn left a long way down the street.
   E Go up the road and take a left turn at the field.

3 What is the best interpretation of the following coded message: A1, G2, G(11), 7

   A The best vehicle to take is the train.
   B The right way to travel is by train.
   C The man must go by train.
   D The correct way for the woman to travel is by train.
   E The woman must stay on the train.

4 What is the best interpretation of the following coded message: G[B(11,9), (G(F))A], C12(4)

   A Follow the laws or be severely punished.
   B In general the rights of people should be firmly respected.
   C It is not rights we need but severe beatings.
   D One rule is in place for a particular group, another rule for a different group.
   E Stay away from illegal activity such as assault.

5 What is the best interpretation of the following coded message: (GC)2, 6, 10

   A The girl laughed at the joke.
   B The man did something funny.
   C The young man made a joke.
   D The smaller lady joked first.
   E Everyone was happy.

6 What would be the best way to encode the following message: The boy saw the smoke

   A (G,C)2, 13, 5
   B B(2), G, 5
   C 9D(5), E(2), 13
   D 11(5), 2(1), 4
   E 1, 2, 13, 5

7 What is the best interpretation of the following coded message: CD, 11, C7

   A The train was moving slower.
   B The small locomotive quickly slowed down.
   C The training session stays last.
   D The big locomotive stayed very slow.
   E Constantly training hard is very tiring.

8 What is the best interpretation of the following coded message: E, 11, G9

   A Keep everything open.
   B Don't close anything.
   C All the things are kept out of reach.
   D Keep the medicines locked away.
   E Everything fell into the hole.

9 Which of the following would be the most useful and the second most useful additions to the codes in order to convey the message accurately? Message: I heard the car strike the sign post.

A Heard
B Car
C Strike
D Sign
E Post

10 What would be the best way to encode the following message: All the people saw the man fall over

A F(E), 6, 2, 1(4)
B E, GF(2), 13, 2, 6(4)
C B(C, E) ,13, C2, C4
D G(11), A(D), 8, 10(8)
E 1, G(2), F(6(4)), 14

11 What is the best interpretation of the following coded message: 14, GD, 7, 12, F3

A I saw the slow train move into the station.
B The train crashed into the tunnel.
C I did not know the train had crashed.
D The particular train that crashed into the slow train was going too fast.
E I heard the fast train crash into the field.

12 Which of the following would be the most useful and the second most useful additions to the codes in order to convey the message accurately? Message: After the journey the man and woman met under the bridge.

A After
B Journey
C Met
D Under
E Bridge

13 What would be the best way to encode the following message: This man met the woman while travelling.

A 2, 11, G2, 12
B F2, B, G2, GF(1)
C G2, C2, E6, 13
D GF(1), F2, 2, 13
E 10, 4, GF(1), 8

New Information Added

General rules	Basic codes
A = right	1 = transport
B = join	2 = man
C = plus	3 = land
D = slow	4 = down
E = total	5 = smoke
F = specific	6 = do
G = opposite	7 = train
	8 = post
	9 = close
	10 = joke
	11 = stay
	12 = strike
	13 = see
	14 = hear

Complex information	Emotions
101 = home	201 = sad
102 = medicine	202 = poor
103 = play	203 = tree
104 = school	204 = heal
105 = learn	205 = ball
106 = help	

14 What is the best interpretation of the following coded message: (GC)2, 14, (2F) 101, 6(5)

  A The boy heard that my house is on fire.
  B The house was full of smoke and no-one could see.
  C I heard that there was smoke in my home.
  D The young lady felt the fire and smelt the smoke.
  E I was told by the boy that the house was smoky.

15 What is the best interpretation of the following coded message: 102, 204, (GF)2, 1, G(201)C, 3

  A The girls went to the hospital to search for the saddest people.
  B When the patients were given the medicine they were made happier.
  C The pills were used to heal the men and women and they took them until they were better.
  D The medicine could not cure the patients and they died.
  E The medicine cured the people and they went to a happier place.

16 What is the best interpretation of the following coded message: 103, GF(102(2), B, 102(G2)) 10

  A The doctors and nurses had fun with us.
  B We played doctors and nurses.
  C We played a joke on the doctors and nurses.
  D The doctors played a joke on the nurses.
  E We played doctors and nurses for fun.

17 What is the best interpretation of the following coded message: 104 G(C2), 6, 12C, 205

    A The boy kicked the ball hard at school.
    B The young school boy played hard ball.
    C The school boy kicked the ball hard.
    D The children at school were not allowed to kick the ball.
    E We like playing football at school.

18 What is the best interpretation of the following coded message: E, 105, G(103), C, 6, 7, 104

    A We learn to work at school but also play.
    B We all learnt to work and train at school.
    C We all learn through playing at school.
    D The whole school can play and do extra training.
    E Stay in school to learn how to work hard.

19 Which of the following would be the most useful and the second most useful additions to the codes in order to convey the message accurately? Message: The puppy was a major hindrance to the mother dog.

    A Puppy
    B Major
    C Hindrance
    D Mother
    E Dog

20 What would be the best way to encode the following message: Help me get out of the tree.

    A 106, 10, 11, 203
    B 106, G2, C4, 202, 3
    C 203, 6, 4, 9, 12, 101
    D F106, G11, 6, 4, 203
    E 106, F, G11, 4, 203

21 What is the best interpretation of the following coded message: 2, G6, G106, 201, GF(GC(2))

    A The man did not help the unhappy children.
    B The people do not help the sad man.
    C The boy wanted to help the other children.
    D The man did not harm the sad children.
    E The man and the children did not feel sadness.

22 Which of the following would be the most useful and the second most useful additions to the codes in order to convey the message accurately? Message: The rich old man was unwell and needed his medication.

A Man
B Medication
C Needed
D Old
E Unwell

23 Which of the following would be the most useful and the second most useful additions to the codes in order to convey the message accurately? Message: The doctor wanted to know how much I smoked and what drugs I had been taking.

A Doctor
B Wanted
C How much
D Drugs
E Taking

24 What would be the best way to encode the following message: The school closed since the tree fell on it.

A 9(104), 11, 203, 4, 5
B 104, 9, F, 203, 12, 4
C G(E)104, E(6), 12, 4, 101
D 14, 2, 9, 104, 12, 13
E 3, B, 104, G(105), G(106)

25 What would be the best way to encode the following message: The unfortunate man could not hear.

A G(201), 2, F14, G6
B 204, 106, 101, 2, G6
C 202, G6, 14
D 202(2), G6, 14
E 11, D, 104, G6, 202, 2

26 What would be the best way to encode the following message: The boy threw the big ball in front of the car.

A GC(2), 12, C205, 6, G, 1
B G2, 6, G205, 6, G1
C 2, 10, 205, C, 1
D F2, F3, C205, 6, G, 7
E 13, 205, G, 1

END OF DECISION ANALYSIS SECTION

END OF PAPER 1

UKCAT PRACTICE QUESTIONS

SAMPLE PAPER 2

Verbal Reasoning – *for full instructions see Sample Paper 1*

Time allowed: 21 minutes

Item 1

China has long been associated with bicycles. Not too long ago China had 500 million bicycles; that is one bicycle for every two people in its population. Bicycles in China are an integral part of every day life and are an important means of transportation. This is quite different from bike riding as a way of physical exercise or as a sport which is the case in the West.

The bicycles used in China are basic; very basic. None come equipped with lights of any kind for night-time riding. Not only are the bicycles used basic, but because many families can only afford one bicycle, they are used to carry loads they were never intended to carry; sometimes carrying up to 3 people at a time. However, this scene tends to vanish with improvement in living standards; When a family is rich enough they can afford two or more bikes.

1 According to the passage, not too long ago the population of China was 1 billion?
2 The bicycles found in the West are more sophisticated than those found in China.
3 Bicycles are an important means of getting around in China.
4 China is unique in its love for bicycles.

Item 2

In the UK one can obtain an estimate of the amount of crime occurring over the previous 12 months from the results of the British Crime Survey (BCS). This is commissioned by the Home Office on a continuous basis, which reports every year and only publishes updates of major areas of crime every quarter. The BCS relies on people's direct experience of crime which is obtained via a questionnaire.

It is considered more authoritative than official police statistics which by definition can only reflect *reported* crime. Since the BCS interviews victims of crime and asks about their own experience of crime, many crimes which victims may consider to be too trivial to report to the police are included. This tends to give a more accurate figure of crime.

The BCS is not totally comprehensive however. It does not include certain crimes committed against children, retail and commercial crime and, significantly, certain violent crimes and homicide.

1 By using official police statistics one can tell how much crime is occurring in a year.
2 All crime updates of the BCS are published every four months.
3 If you wish to know the number of murders committed in a year you cannot rely on the BCS.
4 The BCS obtains its data from interviews of families of the victims of crime.

Item 3

Garlic, a member of the onion family, is well known for its distinctly sharp flavour. This is thought to be a defensive mechanism: the unpleasant taste deterring pests which may otherwise destroy the crop by eating the plant. Interestingly though, the chemicals responsible for the taste are not present until the plant cells have been damaged. Storage vacuoles in the plant cells contain enzymes which react with other innocuous substances in the cell cytoplasm. When the cells are traumatised – by chewing, chopping or crushing – the vacuoles are broken open and the released enzymes can act: thus forming new substances responsible for the flavour. Many sulphur-containing compounds contribute to this flavour, with allicin being the major factor. The enzyme alliinase is present in the vacuoles and this acts on cytoplasmic alliin to form allicin.

Fresh garlic is often more unbearable on the palate than cooked garlic. This is due to the fact that allicin is not very stable; although it gives raw garlic its sharp spiciness, upon cooking allicin is rapidly destroyed and the flavour mellows.

1 Allicin is a chemical present in raw garlic until it is crushed.
2 Vacuoles in garlic contain the enzymes such as alliin.
3 Allicin is a sulphur-containing compound.
4 Cooked garlic is not as flavoursome as raw garlic.

Item 4

The terms WWW or the World Wide Web and the Internet are often (wrongly) used interchangeably. They are not synonymous: the Internet is a collection of interconnected computer networks, linked by some medium that carries information; copper wires, fibre-optic cables, wireless connections, etc.; the Web on the other hand is a collection of interconnected documents and other resources, linked by hyperlinks and URLs. The World Wide Web can be accessed via the Internet, as can many other services including e-mail and file sharing.

A good way to look at these terms is with reference to the Internet protocol suite. The Internet protocol suite can be thought of as a set of layers.

Each layer solves a set of problems involving the transmission of data, and services the needs of the upper layer protocols.

So this collection of standards and protocols is organised into layers such that each layer provides the foundation and the services required by the layer above. The lower layers – which comprise the Internet – therefore form the framework of communication upon which the higher layers – comprising the WWW – can operate.

1 The WWW is associated with the Internet.
2 E-mail and file sharing are similar to the WWW in that they can all be accessed via the Internet.
3 The higher layers of the Internet protocol suite cannot operate without the lower layers.
4 The WWW is made up of resources such as documents.

Item 5

Modern navigation systems are almost exclusively based on satellites and rely on Global Positioning System (GPS) technology. These are of use to aircraft pilots, particularly in military scenarios, as well as mariners and land-based vehicle users, including civilians. The technology utilises a GPS receiver computing its own position relative to several orbiting satellites. Receivers come in many forms – from essential components of fighter jets and transatlantic seafaring tankers to additional features on cars, mobile phones and even watches.

1 All modern navigation systems employ GPS.
2 The GPS systems can be of some benefit to sailors.
3 Without GPS technology, fighter jets would not be fully functional.
4 Most modern watches have GPS technology.

Item 6

A type of strategy board game similar to chess is called mancala. In fact there is no actual game called mancala, more that mancala describes a family of games including Oware (in West Africa), Congklak (in Indonesia) and Kalah (in the United States and Europe). In general there is a "count and capture" game play whereby the playing pieces (also called "seeds") are moved from one hole in the playing board to another (a process aptly known as "sowing"). The player aims to capture their opponents seeds; the process for capturing varies somewhat between games.

Images of mancala games in progress have been found by archaeologists on pottery dating back to the 6th or 7th century in East Africa.

1 Mancala can be played like chess.
2 Kalah is only played in Europe.
3 Seeds are sown in all types of Mancala.
4 Mancala games have been found by archaeologists.

Item 7

In the faculty of divinity, the term of address, "Doctor," is reserved for those who have obtained the degree "Doctor of Divinity" or D.D. at a university or who have received an honorary degree of this kind. Such a member of the church may be addressed as the Reverend Dr Paul Smith or the Reverend Paul Smith D.D.

In the faculty of medicine those who have taken a medical degree lower than M.D. (Doctor of Medicine), e.g. M.B., ChB, are given the courtesy title of Doctor. In the faculty of surgery, surgeons who have taken a fellowship in surgery e.g. FRCS (Fellow of the Royal College of Surgeons) are addressed as Mister or Miss.

1 A person with the title "doctor" may not be medically qualified.
2 For a member of the church to be addressed as "Doctor" it is necessary they have obtained a D.D. degree at university.
3 A surgeon with a medical degree could be addressed as "Mister".
4 Someone with a PhD should use the title "Doctor".

Item 8

The cockroaches most commonly encountered by people in their homes and other places of meeting are the German, the American, and the Oriental cockroaches. These three types of cockroaches can be distinguished by their colour and size. They are nocturnal, remaining hidden during the day and becoming active at night to obtain food and water, and to reproduce.

With the exception of the female Oriental cockroach, the adults of these three cockroaches have well-developed wings. However, they almost never fly; movement by both the adults and the wingless nymphs is by walking or rapid running.

Food, water and places to hide are the three main requirements of cockroaches. Therefore, they found in situations where these requirements can be met. Cockroaches will eat almost anything: left-over human food, toothpaste, milk, sugary materials, glue, soap, faeces, etc.

The German cockroach is usually found in kitchens; the American cockroach appears most commonly in food establishments; and the Oriental cockroach is usually associated with dampness around sinks or in basements. Cockroaches are not normally encountered by man unless their populations become very large.

1 Cockroaches are more active at night.
2 Cockroaches eat faeces.
3 Cockroaches are generally found in dirty environments.
4 With the exception of the Oriental cockroach, most cockroaches almost never fly.

Item 9

Nauru is the world's smallest independent republic with a population of less than 15,000 and a land area of just over 21 km². Located in the South Pacific more than 80% of the island's inhabitants are of Micronesian or Polynesian descent, and the majority are Nauruan.

Throughout its history Nauru has been administered variously by the French, German, UK, New Zealand, Australian and Japanese Governments, but gained independence in 1968. Almost all the countries which ruled over Nauru exploited its natural resource, phosphate. In fact, Nauru is one large phosphate rock. During the 20th century, Nauruans gained great economic wealth, relative to neighbouring islands, from phosphate exports. However, supplies of the mineral are now much depleted and the islanders are paying the price of their rapid economic rise.

Not only has there been much environmental damage left in the wake of phosphate mining but also there are health implications which arose following the islanders increased prosperity: Nauruans are among the most obese in the world and have one of the highest rates of diabetes.

1 The republic of Nauru has been independent for over 35 years.
2 Nauruans are of Micronesian descent.
3 The UK exploited Nauru for its phosphate reserves.
4 Increased levels of diabetes results from increased levels of obesity.

Item 10

There are many ways to define biodiversity, since this concept can be approached from many different angles depending on who is concerned with it. A geneticist may wish to explore the diversity of genes – i.e. mutations occurring at the level of DNA – whilst an ecologist will have a broader view. The ecological paradigm of biodiversity encompasses many disparate species interacting with each other in an ecosystem, and furthermore, the interaction of completely separate ecosystems. Somewhere in the middle of this hierarchical structure there exists the biologist's view of biodiversity which focuses on the organism.

One may try to include the interests of all parties in a definition and consensus has been reached with a definition stating biodiversity is the variability among living organisms from all sources and the ecological complexes of which they are part.

1 Genetic mutation rates are a valid way of defining biodiversity for a geneticist.
2 The concept of biodiversity is empirical and straightforward to define.
3 An ecologist's paradigm of biodiversity focuses solely on separate interactions of an ecosystem.
4 Implicit in a theory of variability of living organisms is the process of evolution by natural selection.

Item 11

It is perhaps hard to believe that common salt – the kind which one freely uses at the dinner table – was once a most valued commodity. Indeed, it is said that as recently as just a few centuries ago salt was the cause of wars, literally making or breaking an empire.

The value of salt can still be seen today, in the English word "salary" which derives from the Latin word "sal", meaning "salt". The Romans, for whom Latin was the native language, would pay their soldiers with salt, so prized was this mineral. Hundreds of years later the French were charging a salt tax known as the gabelle, which was very unpopular and caused smugglers to engage in illicit trading of contraband salt. However taxing salt can be traced back even earlier perhaps to two thousand years ago in Asia.

Not only was the salt of great intrinsic worth, but so too was any food which could be preserved using salt since this could lead to the trading of salted produce over long distances.

1   Salt is still valuable today.
2   The Romans spoke many languages.
3   French smugglers would legally trade in salt to avoid the gabelle.
4   Salted goods were always traded over long distances.

END OF VERBAL REASONING SECTION

Quantitative Reasoning – *for full instructions see Sample Paper 1*

Time allowed: 21 minutes

Item 1

The table below shows the production costs for the first 10,000 units of the concept cars of five leading companies in millions of US dollars.

Car Make	Cost of Production (millions of US dollars)			Retail price (thousands of US dollars)
	Design	Manufacture	Development	
Honda	30	10	60	20
Ford	25	35	40	24
BMW	40	30	50	48
Audi	35	35	35	35
Mercedes	15	60	90	65

1   Which company has the greatest difference between development cost and retail price?

   A Honda
   B Ford
   C BMW
   D Audi
   E Mercedes

2   How much greater (as a percentage) is the largest cost of Manufacture than the smallest cost of Manufacture?

   A 83%
   B 100%
   C 500%
   D 600%
   E Can't tell

3   If there are no additional costs (in addition to production cost), how many cars do Honda have to sell in order to break even?

   A 100,000
   B 500
   C 5,000
   D 50,000
   E 500,000

4 For every 10,000 cars sold, how much more of a profit will BMW make than Honda?

   A $220 million
   B $240 million
   C $260 million
   D $280 million
   E $480 million

Item 2

The chart below shows the total rainfall recorded (in mm) for each month over a year.

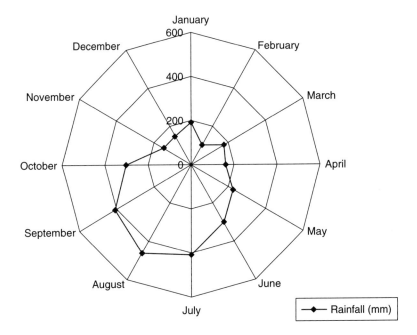

1 Between which of the following months was the greatest difference in monthly rainfall recorded?

   A January–October
   B August–September
   C September–October
   D October–November
   E November–December

2 If the total rainfall was 50% greater in the following year how much rain-fall would you expect there to be in the following January (assuming the relative proportions of monthly rainfall remain the same)?

A 50 mm
B 95 mm
C 240 mm
D 285 mm
E 300 mm

3 If the risk of flooding increases by one percentage point for every 10 mm of rain over 200 mm and the background risk is 8% (below 200 mm) what is the risk of flooding in August?

A 26%
B 27%
C 35%
D 47%
E 60%

4 Five years ago rainfall each month was 50 mm more than the previous month. If it rained 50 mm in January, between which of the following months would there be the smallest percentage increase in rainfall?

A January–February
B February–March
C March–April
D August–October
E August–December

Item 3

The chart below shows the results of a traffic survey. The numbers in each bar show the actual number of vehicles of each colour counted. These are all the types of vehicles considered.

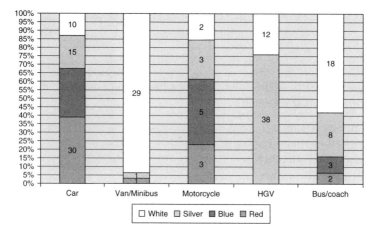

1 What is the approximate ratio of red vehicles to white?

    A 1:2
    B 1:3
    C 3:7
    D 7:20
    E 75:40

2 How many blue cars were counted?

    A 20
    B 22
    C 24
    D 28
    E Can't tell

3 If in the last survey there were 5 less red cars, 1 less red van and 3 less red motorcycles, and no change in the other vehicles which of the following fractions correctly represents the increase in red vehicles from last survey?

    A 1/4
    B 1/3
    C 1/2
    D 3/4
    E 4/3

4 If last year the ratio of Vans:HGVs was 1:3, how many HGVs were counted last year?

    A 10
    B 31
    C 50
    D 93
    E Can't tell

Item 4

The table below shows the results of a survey of the shoe sizes of 300 Males and Females

Shoe size	Male	Female	Shoe size	Male	Female
2	0	5	8	40	8
3	0	6	9	35	4
4	2	16	10	20	2
5	6	46	11	5	0
6	12	30	12	3	0
7	25	33	13	2	0
			Totals:	150	150

1 What was the most common shoe size for Males?

   A 2
   B 4
   C 6
   D 8
   E Can't tell

2 What was the largest range of shoe sizes shown by either group?

   A 7
   B 8
   C 9
   D 10
   E 11

3 The standard prices of Men's and Women's shoes are £76 and £64 respectively. If the price is increased by £2 for every size above size 10, how much would a pair of Men's size 13 shoes cost?

   A £78
   B £80
   C £82
   D £84
   E Can't tell

4 What is the ratio between the number of males and females in the whole group wearing size 6 shoes?

   A 2:5
   B 4:8
   C 12:32
   D 20:3
   E 40:3

Item 5

The table below shows the percentage of the population infected with HIV in certain African countries between the years 1988 and 2003.

Country	1988	1993	1998	2003
Angola	1.5	3.4	3.8	4.5
Botswana	2.3	11.6	25.4	33.4
Central African Republic	3.8	8.9	10.1	10.5
Gambia	0.1	0.2	0.6	0.9
Lesotho	0.9	11.3	22.1	35.8
South Africa	0.8	4.9	15.5	25.6
Uganda	18.8	14.6	9.9	5.1
Zimbabwe	1.1	25.5	30.5	35.4

1 Which country had the most people affected by HIV in 1998?

    A Botswana
    B Gambia
    C South Africa
    D Zimbabwe
    E Can't tell

2 The population of the Central African Republic is twice the population of Lesotho. In which year were there approximately equal numbers of HIV infected individuals in both countries?

    A 1988
    B 1993
    C 1998
    D 2003
    E Can't tell

3 Assuming the population of the country remained static at 12 million from 1988 to 2003 how many more people were infected with HIV in Angola in 2003 compared with 1988?

    A 72,000
    B 180,000
    C 360,000
    D 540,000
    E Can't tell

4 If the population of Uganda was 22 million in 2000 estimate how many people were infected with HIV based on the linear trend shown.

    A 1,056,000
    B 1,122,000
    C 1,760,000
    D 1,924,000
    E 2,200,000

Item 6

The height of 350 plant saplings after the addition of a nutrient is measured at various times over a period of 8 days. The graph below shows the distribution of heights for the whole population excluding the top and bottom 10% of the plants. Each "percentile" graph line represents the height at which a certain percentage of plants have grown to that height.

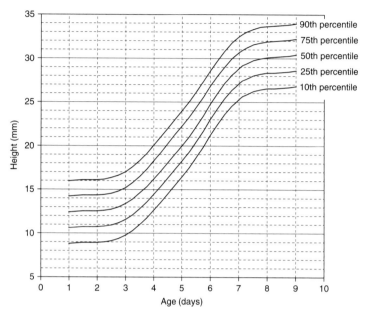

1 How many plants had definitely grown to more than 24 mm by day 5?

   A 0
   B 10
   C 35
   D 90
   E Can't tell

2 Which centile showed the maximum percentage increase in growth over the 8 days?

   A 10th
   B 25th
   C 50th
   D 75th
   E 90th

3 A second nutrient is added at day 3, that causes the growth rate to increase by 50%. What would be the percentage difference between the height of the 90th centile WITHOUT the second nutrient and minimum height achieved by the middle 50% of plants WITH the second nutrient by day 7?

   A 6%
   B 7%
   C 8%
   D 9%
   E 10%

4 If the garden centre specifies a minimum height of 29 mm for purchase at the full price of £1.20 per sapling and the rest are sold at 50p each, what is the approximate difference in profit between selling at day 7 and day 9 (assuming costs remain the same)?

A £55
B £85
C £105
D £145
E £205

Item 7

The travel chart below shows the distances, in miles, between various cities in the USA.

	Chicago	Denver	Houston	Kansas City	Los Angeles	Minneapolis	Miami	New York	San Francisco	Seattle
Atlanta	715	1,405	800	805	2,185	1,135	665	865	2,495	2,785
	Chicago	?	1,085	525	2,020	410	1,380	795	2,135	2,070
		Denver	1,120	600	1,025	915	2,065	1,780	1,270	1,335
			Houston	795	1,550	1,230	1,190	1,635	1,930	2,450
				Kansas City	1,625	440	1,470	1,195	1,865	1,900
					Los Angeles	1,935	2,740	2,800	385	1,140
						Minneapolis	1,795	1,200	2,010	2,015
							Miami	1,280	3,115	3,365
								New York	3,055	2,860
									San Francisco	810

1 What is the distance in miles from Miami to San Francisco via Kansas City?

A 2,335
B 3,248
C 3,335
D 4,585
E Can't tell

2 Assuming the same road connects Atlanta, Chicago and Denver, what is the distance in miles from Denver to Chicago on that road?

A 680
B 690
C 700
D 715
E Can't tell

3 How long will it take for a car travelling at an average speed of 55 miles per hour to travel the quoted distance from New York to Houston?

  A 29 hours 7 minutes
  B 29 hours 32 minutes
  C 29 hours 44 minutes
  D 30 hours 12 minutes
  E Can't tell.

4 If my car travels 40 miles per gallon of petrol and holds a maximum of 10 gallons at a time, how many times shall I need to stop for petrol if I travel a journey the quoted distance from Miami to Kansas City (assuming I start with a full tank)?

  A 2 times
  B 3 times
  C 4 times
  D 5 times
  E Can't tell

Item 8

The following chart is an analysis of the Earth's outer crust, by Element.

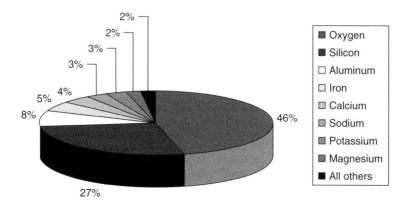

1 Which element comprises the biggest share of the Earth's outer crust?

  A Oxygen
  B Silicon
  C Aluminium
  D Iron
  E Calcium

2 Which of the following pairs of elements together form the largest share shown in the graph?

  A Magnesium and Calcium
  B Magnesium and Sodium
  C Magnesium and Aluminium
  D Calcium and Iron
  E Calcium and Aluminium

3 If the Earth's mass is 6×10^{24} kg what is the mass of Iron making up the crust?

  A 3×10^{23}
  B 3×10^{24}
  C 6×10^{23}
  D 6×10^{24}
  E Can't tell

4 If all the Calcium were replaced by Sodium, what would be the mass of Sodium in the Earth's outer crust?

  A 42×10^{22}
  B 42×10^{23}
  C 18×10^{22}
  D 1.8×10^{24}
  E Can't tell

Item 9

The table below records the properties of various metals.

Material	Resistivity ($\times 10^{-8}$) (Ωm)	Conductivity ($\times 10^{7}$) (Ω^{-1}m^{-1})
Silver	1.59	6.97
Copper	1.68	5.95
Aluminium	2.65	3.55
Tungsten	6.71	1.93
Iron	9.71	1.03
Platinum	10.63	0.94
Lead	22	0.45
Mercury	98	0.14

1 How many times more resistive is Iron than Aluminium?

  A 0.27
  B 0.29
  C 0.34
  D 3.7
  E 3.5

2 Between which of the following metals is there the greatest difference in conductivity?

   A Silver and Platinum
   B Copper and Mercury
   C Aluminium and Platinum
   D Iron and Mercury
   E Lead and Tungsten

3 The conductivity of which of the following materials has a value approximately 1/3 the value of the resistivity of Lead?

   A Silver
   B Copper
   C Tungsten
   D Mercury
   E Can't tell

4 If Resistance (in ohms) is calculated as (Resistivity × Length (in metres))/ Area (in square metres), what would be the resistance of a 10 cm copper wire with a cross-sectional area of 0.000004 square metres?

   A 42 ohms
   B 4.2 ohms
   C 0.42 ohms
   D 0.0042 ohms
   E 0.00042 ohms

Item 10

The table below shows the area, capitals and population of 6 countries, compared to that of the world.

Country	Capital city	Area (sq. km)	2002 population estimate
Nigeria	Abuja	923,768	129,934,911
United Kingdom	London	244,820	59,778,002
Ecuador	Quito	283,560	13,447,494
Tajikistan	Dushanbe	143,100	6,719,567
Canada	Ottawa	9,976,140	31,902,268
Sri Lanka	Colombo	65,610	19,576,783
World	–	510,072,000	6,233,821,945

1 Which of the countries in the table shown above hold the largest share of the world's population?

   A Nigeria
   B United Kingdom
   C Ecuador
   D Tajikistan
   E Canada

2 Which country from the six listed in the table has the largest population density?

   A United Kingdom
   B Tajikistan
   C Canada
   D Sri Lanka
   E Ecuador

3 How many countries from the table have a population density smaller than the average population density (of the countries listed in the table)?

   A 1
   B 2
   C 3
   D 4
   E 5

4 How many countries the size of Canada could completely fit onto the Earth's surface?

   A 50
   B 51
   C 52
   D 53
   E 54

END OF QUANTITATIVE REASONING SECTION

Abstract Reasoning – *for full instructions see Sample Paper 1*

Time allowed: 15 minutes

Item 1

Set A	Set B	Test shape 1	Test shape 2	Test shape 3

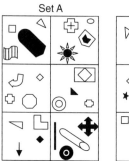
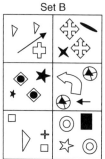
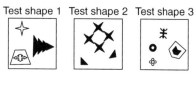

Test shape 4	Test shape 5

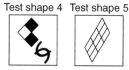

Item 2

Set A	Set B	Test shape 1	Test shape 2	Test shape 3

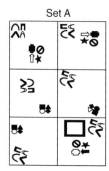
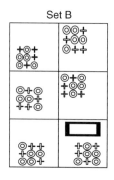
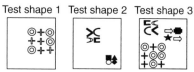

Test shape 4	Test shape 5

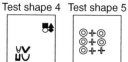

Item 3

Set A	Set B	Test shape 1	Test shape 2	Test shape 3

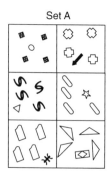
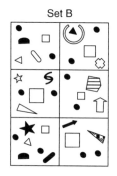
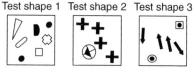

Test shape 4	Test shape 5

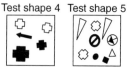

Item 4

Set A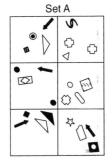

Set B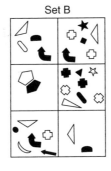

Test shape 1   Test shape 2   Test shape 3
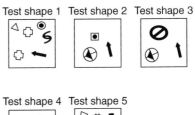

Test shape 4   Test shape 5

Item 5

Set A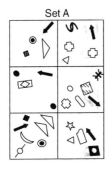

Set B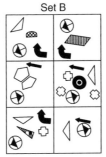

Test shape 1   Test shape 2   Test shape 3

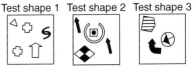

Test shape 4   Test shape 5
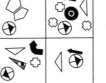

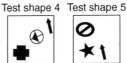

Item 6

Set A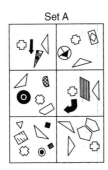

Set B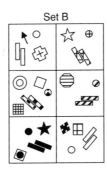

Test shape 1   Test shape 2   Test shape 3

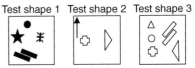

Test shape 4   Test shape 5
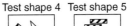

Item 7

Set A 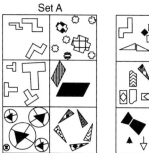 Set B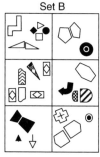

Test shape 1 Test shape 2 Test shape 3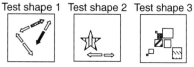

Test shape 4 Test shape 5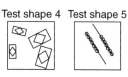

Item 8

Set A 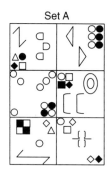 Set B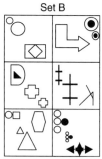

Test shape 1 Test shape 2 Test shape 3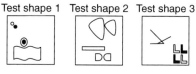

Test shape 4 Test shape 5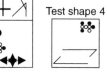

Item 9

Set A 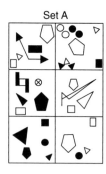 Set B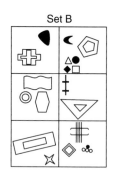

Test shape 1 Test shape 2 Test shape 3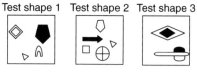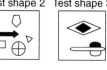

Test shape 4 Test shape 5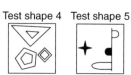

Item 10

Set A

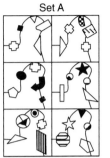

Set B

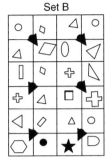

Test shape 1

Test shape 2

Test shape 3

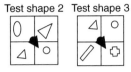

Test shape 4   Test shape 5

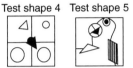

Item 11

Set A

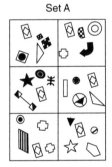

Set B

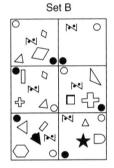

Test shape 1

Test shape 2   Test shape 3

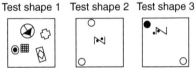

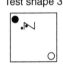

Test shape 4   Test shape 5

Item 12

Set A

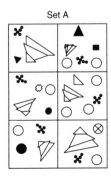

Set B

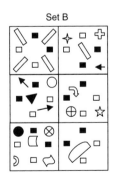

Test shape 1   Test shape 2   Test shape 3

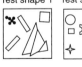

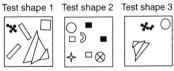

Test shape 4   Test shape 5

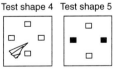

Item 13

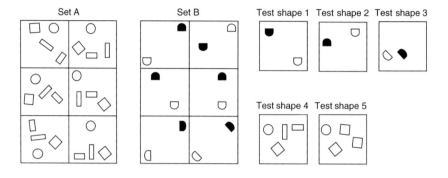

END OF ABSTRACT REASONING SECTION

Decision Analysis – *for full instructions see Sample Paper 1*

Time allowed: 29 minutes

Table of codes

Specific Information	Qualifiers
1 = meeting	A = increase
2 = attack	B = opposite
3 = shipment	C = fast
4 = soldiers	D = generalise
5 = headquarters	E = combine
6 = supply	F = urgent
7 = front line	G = negative
8 = ammunitions	H = more
9 = rations	U = unknown
10 = road	Nx = number = x
11 = land	T = time
12 = sea	
13 = air	
14 = artillery	
15 = enemy	

1 What is the best interpretation of the following coded message: 2, 14, 7

   A Emergency meeting in 4 hours. Alert generals.
   B Enemy fire on front line.
   C Artillery attack increasing on the front line.
   D Attack the munitions factory with extra artillery at the front line.
   E Artillery attack on the front line.

2 What is the best interpretation of the following coded message: 15, B(E), 7

   A Front line combined attack against enemy.
   B Enemy dispersed at front line.
   C Enemy oppose the meeting attempt on front line.
   D Enemy not willing to enter negotiations.
   E Enemy attack quelled on front line.

3 What is the best interpretation of the following coded message: 15(13, 2), T(N12)

   A Attack by air the enemy in 12 hours.
   B Air attack in 12 hours – respond urgently.
   C Enemy air raid in 12 hours.
   D Fly to meet enemy aircraft for 12 hour negotiations.
   E Aircraft carrier spotted in enemy territory 12 hours ago.

4 What is the best interpretation of the following coded message: 6, 9, B(C)

   A Supply more rations as soon as possible.
   B The ration supply has slowed down.
   C Enemy attack on ration supply.
   D Supply less rations.
   E Supply the rations quickly.

5 What would be the best way to encode the following message: Shipments by sea increased less than supplies by land

   A (3,12), B(H), 6(11)3
   B D(3,12) A(H), 6(11)3
   C 10(D12), D6, (3,11)A(B)
   D (3,12), A(B(H)), 6(3,11)
   E D(3,12), B(H), 6(11)

6 Which of the following would be the most useful and the second most useful additions to the codes in order to convey the message accurately? Message: Road blocks operating near front line. All known soldiers must show identification.

   A Identification
   B Known
   C Near
   D Operate
   E Road block

7 What is the best interpretation of the following coded message: H(2,13), T0.

   A More time needed to quell enemy fire power.
   B Make air attacks immediately.
   C More enemy air raids imminent.
   D Further enemy air attack. Await instructions.
   E Extra air patrol reinforcements ordered now.

8 Which of the following would be the most useful and the second most useful additions to the codes in order to convey the message accurately? Message: Unidentified flying object detected 25 miles away.

   A Away
   B Detect
   C Fly
   D Mile
   E Object

9 What would be the best way to encode the following message: Soldiers fighting on the battle ground work together to kill the enemy.

A 4, 2, D7, E, H(2), 15
B 2, 7, H, U(T12), G(C)
C 4, E, 2, 15, H(15)
D 11, 8, 6, 3, 4, 8(GT)
E D7, E, 2, H(15)

10 Which of the following would be the most useful and the second most useful additions to the codes in order to convey the message accurately? Message: All soldiers must defend to the death the emperor's palace.

A Death
B Defend
C Emperor
D Palace
E Soldiers

11 What is the best interpretation of the following coded message: 3(8,9), B(C)A.

A Air supplies of food and medical equipment slowly increasing.
B Rations low. Need supply from reinforcements to increase.
C Ammunitions and ration supply is slowing down.
D Weapons and food supply low. Extra required.
E Ammunition and ration supply quickly decreasing.

12 What is the best interpretation of the following coded message: 2, 15(11,12,13), TN12, BA(7).

A D(101), 2(15), (10,6), H004, 101
B (11,6)2, 101, 004, H(E106)
C 008, 101, 2(15(11,6), B(004), D(E), 4)
D 101, 2(15 (11,6)), B(H) 004, D(101)
E 102, 105, 106, 101, 3, 11, 6

New Information Added

Table of codes

Specific information		Qualifiers	
1 = meeting	9 = rations	A = increase	U = unknown
2 = attack	10 = road	B = opposite	Nx = number = x
3 = shipment	11 = land	C = fast	T = time
4 = soldiers	12 = sea	D = generalise	
5 = headquarters	13 = air	E = combine	
6 = supply	14 = artillery	F = urgent	
7 = front line	15 = enemy	G = negative	
8 = ammunitions		H = more	

Relating to your mission	Danger level/difficulty
101 = mission	004 = mild/easily achievable
102 = danger	005 = moderate/usual precautions
103 = open	006 = severe/full precautions
104 = close	007 = impossible/likely fatal
105 = high	008 = danger to mission/do not attempt
106 = intercept	

13 What would be the best way to encode the following message: The mission to attack enemy land supplies was less easily achievable than the other missions.

   A Attack the enemy by all means in 12 hours. Take troops from the front line.
   B Decrease numbers on the front line. Enemy attack in 12 days by air, sea and land.
   C 12 hours until front line troops attacked by enemy. Expect land, air and sea offensive.
   D Attack the enemy on all fronts. Take 12 divisions from the front line.
   E 12th armoured brigade attacked on front line. Enemy routed by air, sea and land.

14 What would be the best way to encode the following message: Urgent mission at front line but straightforward.

   A F! 101(7), 004
   B F101, D(7), B(006)
   C 103, 101, F(7), B(006)
   D 10, F, D(F), 101 7, 004
   E B(F), 101, 7, B(004)

15 What is the best interpretation of the following coded message: 102 (6, (7)).

   A Danger to mission at front line.
   B Supply in danger. Front line troops to escort.
   C Supply safe. Front line in danger.
   D Supply from front line endangered.
   E Supply for front line troops attacked by enemy.

16 What is the best interpretation of the following coded message: 101(106), 15 (13,2), 006.

   A Attack mission by air. Enemy air attack. Take full precautions.
   B Take full precautions to intercept the enemy by air.
   C Attack the enemy and intercept the attack. Take full precautions.
   D Usual precautions – severe danger. Urgent intercept of enemy by air.
   E Intercept mission. Take full precautions. Enemy air attack.

17 What is the best interpretation of the following coded message: D(102), 105, D(10), H(005).

    A Increased level of danger to road supplies.
    B General danger on high roads, take usual precautions.
    C High level of danger on roads. Take extra precautions.
    D Much danger intercepted on road. Take care.
    E More than moderate precaution required on road.

18 What is the best interpretation of the following coded message: C(2, E, 15(13, 12, 11)), GD(106), G(8), F008.

    A Quick combined enemy air, sea and land assault. No artillery fire power available to intercept. Abandon.
    B Fast enemy combined air, sea and land attack. No ammunitions supply. Priority intercept and abandon.
    C Attack enemy by air, sea and land assault. No artillery fire power. Urgently abandon.
    D Attack enemy by air, land and sea urgently. Do not attempt mission to intercept ammunitions.
    E Do not attempt to intercept enemy combined air, sea and land attack. Abandon urgently.

19 Which of the following would be the most useful and the second most useful additions to the codes in order to convey the message accurately? Message: New order from base: urgent! Try a secret mission not more dangerous missions.

    A Base
    B Order
    C Secret
    D New
    E Try

20 What is the best interpretation of the following coded message: 7(4), (H(G),102), 106, 15, H(C)

    A Front line soldiers in danger of attack. Make an intercept of the enemy.
    B Intercept the enemy now. Dangerous enemy will attack sooner.
    C Soldiers at the front line in graver danger – intercept enemy faster.
    D More danger exists at the front line. Soldiers must intercept the enemy.
    E More soldiers on the front line in extreme danger. Intercept the enemy fast.

21 What would be the best way to encode the following message: Urgent: intercept enemy ammunitions supply.

   A F!, 106, 15(H,6), 8
   B F!, 104, H(T)
   C F(106), 5(15), 6(7), 8
   D F, 15(6,8), 106
   E B(F), 007, H(G), E(6,8) 106

22 What is the best interpretation of the following coded message: 3(6), E(8,9), 104(10), A(B,C) 6(7), T(N22).

   A Ammunition and rations shipment more delayed due to road closure – will arrive in 22 hours.
   B Shipment of ammunition and rations supply delayed more by road closure. Will supply front line in 22 hours.
   C Ammunition and rations supply will arrive late due to road block. Will reach front line 22 hours later.
   D Shipment and combined supply of ammunition will reach front line in 22 hours.
   E Road blocks delayed the speed of the mission. 22 hour delay in front line restocking.

23 Which of the following would be the most useful and the second most useful additions to the codes in order to convey the message accurately? Message: Halt all supplies. Otherwise likely fatal disaster to front line troops.

   A All
   B Disaster
   C Halt
   D Otherwise
   E Supplies

24 What would be the best way to encode the following message: Usual precautions for mission, but not urgent.

   A 005, 101, G(F)
   B 005, 101, F
   C G(005), 101, F
   D D(005), U101, B(F)
   E 005, B101, GF

25 What is the best interpretation of the following coded message: T(104,11), 2(12)006, 15(14), 2CE(10,11).

   A In 104 hours by land, a severe attack by sea will occur. Enemy artillery will attack by land and road.

   B On nearing land, a sea attack would be too dangerous due to enemy artillery fire, therefore use a fast invasion by land.

   C A land attack would be more dangerous than sea attack for enemy artillery fire to be drawn to the land occurs faster.

   D Time spent closer to land is too dangerous. Fire on enemy land quickly.

   E A land assault faster than the enemy artillery can fire on us is less dangerous than by sea.

26 What would be the best way to encode the following message: Easy mission: no danger from enemy currently – attack as quickly as possible.

   A 004, 101, G(102(15)), 2, G(C,D)

   B 101 (004), B(102)(15), 2A

   C (101)G(004), B(102)(15), (2)(D)(C)

   D 101, 104, B102(2), 15, D(C)

   E 004 (101), G(102)(15), 2, D(C)

END OF DECISION ANALYSIS SECTION
END OF PAPER 2

9
Solutions

Chapter 1 – Quantitative analysis

Quick Test 3	
1	Can't tell from given information
2	0.42%
3	~4% increase
Quick Test 5	
1	9 hours 9 minutes
2	11 hours 49 minutes
3	1.5 cm
4	108°
Quick Test 6	
1	5
2	June 1995
3A	No – cannot have 84 seconds
3B	Yes
3C	No – 60 seconds = 1 minute on a clock
3D	Cannot have 28 hours on a clock
4	Thursday
5	50
6	2 (March and November)
Quick Test 8	
1	8
2a	minimum = 1 (1p, 2p, 5p or 10p)
2b	maximum = 6 (1p, 2p, 5p, 10p, 20p and 50p)
3	2 (20p and 50p)
4	Can't tell (depends on when exactly the conversion is made)
5	Relative to the £, it is a 13% reduction (not 15%)
6	$143.68
7	21% (21p in the £)
Quick Test 11	
1	Yes
2	Yes
Quick Test 13	
1	A, B, C, D (all correct)

Part C: Practice	
Question	Answer
1	D
2	B
3	D
4	£1.39
5	E
6	C
7	C
8	B
9	A
10	E
11	E
12	(i) 1.08 seconds (ii) 7 in total
13	24/55

Chapter 2 – Critical analysis

Part C: Practice				
Question	Answer			
2	E			
3	A			
4	A			
5	E			
6	A and E			
7	D			
8	A, C and F			
9	E and F			
10	B and C			
11	A			
12	A			
16	C	C	C	A
17	A	A	A	A
18	C	A	A	C
19	C	C	B	C
20	B	C	A	A
21	A	B	A	B

Chapter 3 – Scientific knowledge and application

Part C: Practice	
Question	Answer
1*	A – A; B – A; C – A; D – A; E – C
2*	i – C; ii – B; iii – D
3	B
4*	D, A, G, I, B, C or F
5	A
6	A
7	iv
8	50%
9	A
10*	i – E; ii – D; iii – B
11	B
12	A
13*	i – D; ii – A or H; iii – E; iv – G; v – H or C; vi – C or H
14*	A – v; B – iv; C – vii; D – vi; E – i
15*	p – 6; q – 3; r – 2; s – 4
16*	A – i; B – iv; C – iii; D – ii;
17	A
18	B
19	A
20	50
21	A
22	0.75
23	2 m to left OR 2 m to right
24	A
25	B
26	D
27*	A, B, C
28	9.7
29*	A and C
30	D
31	B
32	A
33	E
*All answers must be correct in order to score 1 point	

Chapter 7 – BMAT practice papers

PAPER A (maximum score 62)

SECTION 1	
Question	Answer
1	C
2	C
3	C
4	E
5	D
6	D
7	C
8	D
9	A
10*	A and C
11	B
12	D
13	C
14	C
15	E
16	C
17	C
18	E
19	B
20	D
21	B
22	C
23	D
24	D
25	C
26	D
27	£4,920
28	A
29	D
30	D
21	E
32	B
33	A
34	0.6%
35	10%
*All answers must be correct in order to score 1 point	
Maximum Score 35	

SECTION 2	
Question	Answer
1	D
2	9
3*	**a** = **b** = 3
4	C
5	C
6	118
7	A
8*	**a** = 2 **b** = 11
9*	**i** = F **ii** = C **iii** = A
10*	**i** = A **ii** = B **iii** = E **iv** = C
11*	**i** = C **ii** = E **iii** = D **iv** = A **v** = B
12	B
13	D
14	D
15	B
16	C
17	1:3
18	1.3175
19	0.654498 or 55/84
20	D
21*	**a** = 4 **b** = 5 **c** = 4 **d** = 6
22	A
23	C
24*	**i** = C **ii** = B **iii** = A
25	D
26	C
27	D
*All answers must be correct in order to score 1 point	
Maximum Score 27	

PAPER B (maximum score 62)

SECTION 1	
Question	Answer
1	C
2	C
3	D
4*	B and F
5	E
6	B
7	A
8	B
9	C
10	B
11	E
12	D
13	C
14*	B and C
15	B
16	B
17*	C and F
18	D
19	D
20	C
21	D
22	B
23	0.06
24	D
25	D
26	D
27	1 :2 :1
28	C
29	D
30	C
31	E
32	C
33	E
34	E
35*	B, C and D
All answers must be correct in order to score 1 point	
Maximum Score 35	

SECTION 2	
Question	Answer
1	A
2	A
3*	A and C
4*	i = C ii = B iii = A iv = D v = D
5	E
6	A
7	B
8*	A, B, C and D
9	3.33Ω
10	D
11	C
12	B
13	D
14	E
15	E
16	4:1:4:16
17	0.125
18	E
19	E
20*	A, C and D
21*	$p = 5; q = -2$
22	C and E
23	E
24	13.50
25*	B and D
26	C
27	C
*All answers must be correct in order to score 1 point	
Maximum Score 27	

Chapter 8 – UKCAT practice papers

Paper 1 (maximum score 175)

Verbal Reasoning				
Item	Question			
	1	2	3	4
1	B	C	C	B
2	B	C	A	C
3	C	A	C	C
4	C	C	C	C
5	C	C	C	A
6	B	C	A	C
7	B	C	C	C
8	A	A	C	A
9	A	C	B	C
10	C	C	C	A
11	C	A	A	C
Maximum Score 44				

Quantitative Reasoning				
Item	Question			
	1	2	3	4
1	E	E	D	D
2	E	D	E	B
3	E	A	A	D
4	B	C	C	B
5	E	C	D	D
6	A	E	E	D
7	B	A	C	A
8	E	E	B	B
9	B	E	D	E
10	B	A	A	A
Maximum Score 40				

Abstract Reasoning					
Item	Test Shape				
	1	2	3	4	5
1	A	B	A	C	C
2	B	C	C	C	C
3	C	C	A	B	C
4	B	C	A	A	C
5	C	C	C	A	C
6	C	C	C	C	C
7	C	C	B	B	C
8	A	C	A	C	B
9	C	C	C	B	C
10	C	C	A	B	B
11	C	A	B	B	C
12	C	B	B	A	C
13	C	A	B	A	C
Maximum Score 65					

Decision Analysis	
Question	Answer
1	B
2	D
3	D
4	A
5	C
6	A
7	D
8	A
9*	B and D
10	B
11	E
12*	B and E
13	B
14	A
15	E
16	C
17	C
18	B
19*	D and E
20	E
21	D
22*	A and D
23*	B and C
24	B
25	D
26	A
*Both answers must be correct in order to score 1 point	
Maximum Score 26	

Paper 2 (maximum score 175)

Verbal Reasoning				
Item	Question			
	1	2	3	4
1	A	C	A	C
2	B	B	A	B
3	B	B	A	A
4	A	A	A	A
5	C	A	A	C
6	C	B	C	C
7	A	B	A	C
8	C	A	C	C
9	A	A	C	C
10	C	B	B	C
11	C	C	B	C
Maximum Score 44				

Quantitative Reasoning				
Item	Question			
	1	2	3	4
1	E	C	C	C
2	D	E	C	D
3	A	E	B	E
4	D	C	C	A
5	E	E	C	C
6	C	A	C	A
7	C	B	C	B
8	A	E	E	E
9	D	A	E	E
10	A	D	C	B
Maximum Score 40				

Abstract Reasoning					
Item	Test Shape				
	1	2	3	4	5
1	C	C	A	C	C
2	C	C	C	A	B
3	B	A	C	C	C
4	C	C	C	A	C
5	C	C	B	A	A
6	B	C	C	A	B
7	C	B	C	A	A
8	A	B	A	A	C
9	C	A	C	C	C
10	C	C	B	C	C
11	A	C	C	C	C
12	A	B	C	C	C
13	C	C	B	A	C
Maximum Score 65					

Decision Analysis	
Question	Answer
1	E
2	B
3	C
4	B
5	D
6*	A and D
7	C
8*	B and D
9	A
10*	A and C
11	C
12	D
13	B
14	A
15	D
16	E
17	C
18	A
19*	D and E
20	C
21	D
22	B
23*	B and D
24	A
25	B
26	E
*Both answers must be correct in order to score 1 point	
Maximum Score 26	

Index